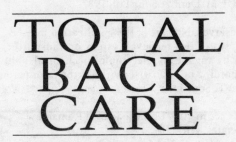

HE LTH
RIGHT

TOTAL
BACK
CARE

Christopher R. Hayne

Foreword by Ruth E. M. Bowden
Professor of Anatomy,
Royal College of Surgeons of England

J. M. Dent & Sons Ltd
London and Melbourne

iv

First published 1987
© Christopher R. Hayne 1987
© Foreword, J. M. Dent & Sons Ltd, 1987

This book is set in 10½/12pt Mediaeval Roman by
AKM Associates (UK) Ltd,
Ajmal House, Hayes Road, Southall, London
Printed in Great Britain by
Guernsey Press Co. Ltd, Guernsey C.I., for
J. M. Dent & Sons Ltd
Aldine House, 33 Welbeck Street, London W1M 8LX

British Library Cataloguing in Publication Data

Hayne, Christopher R.
   Total back care. —— (Healthright)
   1. Backache —— Treatment
   I. Title   II. Series
   616.7'306   RD768

   ISBN 0-460-02439-6

TOTAL
BACK
CARE

About This Book

Back pain, as those who suffer or have suffered know, is a totally individual experience which cannot be shared with any other person. No matter how helpful others may try to be, it is a fact that they cannot feel your pain – and their experiences, either at first or second hand, may only serve to aggravate the situation. When it comes to finding a cure, the conflicting advice so freely provided can add a headache to your back pain!

It is not, perhaps, as readily appreciated that often the cure lies within the power of the sufferer. This book seeks to clarify many of the confusing elements of problems with the back, and then to give information about the various resources which are available to you in seeking your own personal solution. In a number of cases it is possible to do this on a self-help basis, although there will always be problems which are more serious and will require outside assistance of one kind or another.

But back pain *can* in many instances be cured, and recurrences can be prevented. The aim of this book is to enable you both to find an appropriate solution to your particular problem, and to remain free from pain in the future.

Contents

Foreword by Professor Ruth E. M. Bowden ix
Preface xi

1 Backs and Back Pain 1
2 Common Types and Causes of Back Pain 18
3 Self-Help and Self-Assessment 32
4 Standing and Lifting 44
5 Sitting Pretty 57
6 Sleep and Relaxation 66
7 Exercise and Back Pain 80
8 Seeking Medical Help 95
9 Further Help for Back Pain 108
10 Manipulative Therapy 122

To Sum Up . . . 131
Resource List 133
Book List 137
Index 141

Foreword

This small book, written in simple everyday language deserves a large readership. Those enduring the miseries of acute or chronic pain in the back will find advice on what to do in the short and long term. There are very clear indications of when it is necessary to seek professional advice and abandon the 'do-it-yourself' approach to treatment. The few who will ultimately need to have elaborate investigations and even surgical treatment, have straightforward explanations of the tests and of the immediate post-operative care and the process of rehabilitation. This should reduce the fear of the unknown. Patients are reluctant to ask questions and unfortunately some doctors do not explain procedures in simple terms. Both factors add unnecessarily to tension and anxiety and may aggravate the pain and discomfort.

Those who have escaped the experience of trouble with the back, as well as victims, will benefit from the account of the healthy spine, the controlling mechanisms and the changes due to advancing age. Understanding the strengths and weaknesses of the back and acquiring safe techniques of lifting weights all contribute to prevention of damage.

This practical book stems from the author's observant and most thoughtful work as a physiotherapist in hospitals and in industry. He aims not only to treat painful backs, but also, perhaps more importantly, to prevent strain and damage. 'Prevention is better than cure' is certainly true of injuries to the back.

Ruth E. M. Bowden

Preface

When it was first suggested that I might write a book on back pain, I had no idea of the magnitude or complexity of the task I had undertaken. When examined in minute detail, the spine and its associated structures are so intricate that it is easy for the picture to become completely bewildering. My aim has therefore been to provide a clear, simplified account of the way the spine functions and of the wide variety of factors that can produce back pain. If as a result I have been in any way inaccurate from a strictly anatomical or physiological viewpoint, the errors are of course mine.

Anyone who writes a book on back pain relies heavily on the views and experiences of others. A list of the texts that I have drawn on is given at the end of this volume, and may be a useful guide for those who wish to read further on the subject.

I should like to acknowledge with particular gratitude the time, encouragement and constructive advice given to me by Professor Ruth E. M. Bowden. It was due to Professor Bowden and the members of the Back Pain Association Education Committee that I became more involved in the prevention and treatment of this problem. Thanks are also due to my friends and colleagues who have helped me, sometimes unknowingly, to formulate the ideas expressed here. Finally this book would never have been published but for the efforts of my editor, Jocelyn Burton, who spent many hours in the revision of the draft material into its final form.

I hope this book will help you, the reader, in your search

for relief from pain. Having experienced the miseries of back pain myself, I write as a sufferer as well as a therapist committed to the resolution and prevention of this age-old problem.

1987   Christopher R. Hayne

To my wife Jean, who has patiently borne with my involvement with back pain for many years

1   *Backs and Back Pain*

When an attack of back pain occurs, it is natural to react with anxiety, particularly if you have had previous similar experiences. Some basic information about back pain may at least help to alleviate the initial distress and confusion.

In the middle of an episode of back pain you may feel that life will never be normal again. It may nevertheless console you to know that your experience is not unique, and that for many sufferers the pain is of relatively short duration. Each year in Britain some 1.5 million people seek the assistance of their doctors because of back pain. In addition, a large number choose alternative therapy from osteopaths, chiropractors and acupuncturists. For the majority the pain persists for only a few days or weeks. Seventy per cent are better in a month and a further 20 per cent are well on the way to recovery within three months. Less than a quarter of one per cent have to be treated surgically. (All this, of course, may seem rather cold comfort when one day of unspeakable agony is enough.)

Unfortunately, the remaining 10 per cent may have trouble for many months. Even then, however, there are several ways of reducing and alleviating chronic back pain. Simply understanding the cause tends in itself to bring a degree of relief and to reduce the anxiety and tension which aggravate muscular spasm and pain.

What Is Back Pain?

Most patients with back pain are told that they have lumbago, sciatica or a slipped disc, and the treatment is often concentrated on relieving the pain. ('Go to bed and rest', 'Take two tablets every four hours', and so on.) In most cases this treatment works.

However, the terms used by the medical profession often

simply describe a particular set of symptoms, while the underlying cause remains unidentified. Today, more is known about the normal structure and function of the spine than at any other time, but it seems that although our knowledge increases, understanding of the causes of back pain and the design of effective treatment are as elusive as ever. There may therefore be some benefit in a much broader approach.

If you are a typical sufferer, it is most likely that your pain has been caused by some form of mechanical disturbance to the complicated spinal system. Something may have been stretched, torn, squashed or slightly displaced, causing the complex network of pain receptors, which serve the spine, to be stimulated. The pain receptors then send signals to the brain to indicate that something is wrong in a particular area. These nerve impulses also initiate local protective reflex muscle spasm, which could be likened to a do-it-yourself system of splintage. However, excessive and persistent muscle spasm is counterproductive.

In a small percentage of sufferers the cause is not initially mechanical but due to inflammatory processes, not always understood. In such cases the pain may not be restricted to a particular area but can be widespread, varying in location and intensity. In these circumstances, the onset of the pain is often spontaneous, with no history of injury or evidence of mechanical cause. Specialist advice should be sought from a consultant rheumatologist or surgeon if you or your doctor suspect that you are one of the 4 per cent of people who fall into this category. Anti-inflammatory drugs are usually very effective and the problem is not helped permanently by physical treatment.

The majority of cases of back pain which have arisen from other causes present with classical symptoms, easily identified by your doctor. Among these conditions are kidney stones, inflammation of the gall bladder, as well as gynaecological problems or even worry and depression. In the last two instances, some degree of mechanical disorder may be present but pain is magnified by other factors.

Mechanical causes of back pain can be as simple as effects of cold, poor posture or over-use of muscles. The problem becomes more complicated when the muscle fibres are torn, especially if this is accompanied by damage to associated ligaments and tendons. If ligaments themselves are torn or stretched, then the joints are less protected. This can accelerate the wear and tear that occurs as a part of the normal ageing process.

Already various structures have been mentioned, and without some idea of the complex construction and function of the total spinal system it will become increasingly difficult to grasp the underlying principles of cause, prevention and treatment. The anatomy, physiology and biomechanics will be kept here to basic facts, and will avoid any mystifying medical jargon. We can then go on to deal with the various types of back problems in more detail in the chapter which follows.

The Spine – A General View

The spine has evolved into its present form during millions of years. Mechanically, it fulfils a number of different functions:

- It provides the central support necessary to maintain an upright posture. This is vital to a lifestyle in which the upper limbs are used as very special manipulative tools, rather than as a pair of front legs.
- It protects the vital but vulnerable spinal cord and roots of nerves.
- It is flexible enough to permit a wide range of movements, yet has the strength to prevent excessive damage.
- It connects the head, shoulder girdle, pelvis and legs and suspends the upper limbs and rib cage.

Unlike the lower limbs which are made up of two long bones, the femur and the tibia, powered by strong muscles, the spinal column is made up of a number of small bones, the vertebrae. The neck, chest and lower back, although identified as specific areas, are parts of a total structure whose components are interdependent, and anything that happens in one area will almost certainly be reflected in other parts of the spine.

There are 33 vertebrae in the spinal column. The first two, called the atlas and the axis, are specially developed to connect the spine with the base of the skull and also to permit movements of the head on the neck. At the lower end of the spine the last four vertebrae are what remains of the tail in man, and above these are five fused vertebrae which form a flattened triangular segment called the sacrum. The sacrum forms an important part of the pelvic girdle, which links the trunk and lower limbs. The vertebrae from the second to twenty-fourth are separated at the front by specialized pads called the intervertebral discs. At the back there are paired joints: these are small versions of the kind found in the limbs. Their shape governs the direction of possible movement. Both the vertebrae and discs will be discussed more fully a little later on.

Individually, the component parts of the spine are relatively weak, but when combined together they are capable of resisting considerable force. Being a living organism, the spinal column will respond to the stresses and strains that are applied to it by adapting its structure and even shape. In addition, it will undergo a series of progressive degenerative changes as part of the natural process of ageing.

When the normal spine is viewed from the front or back it usually appears to be in a straight line, broadening from the head to the pelvis as the load it carries gets heavier. From the side, however, the spine of an adult in the prime of life resembles an elongated flattened S-shaped mast. The concave curves of the neck and of the lumbar region, or loin, face backwards, while in the chest and pelvis they face forwards. The spine of the neck and loin is very mobile. Rotation is the one free movement in most of the region of the chest, and as might be expected, the pelvis makes a strong girdle with minimal movement. (Mobility increases slightly in women during pregnancy to allow a little more

The spinal column

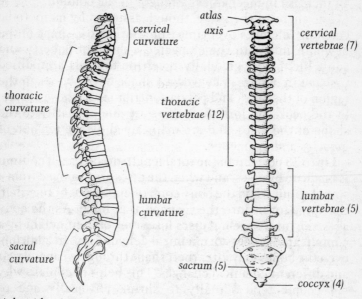

cervical curvature

thoracic curvature

lumbar curvature

sacral curvature

Right side view

atlas
axis

cervical vertebrae (7)

thoracic vertebrae (12)

lumbar vertebrae (5)

sacrum (5)
coccyx (4)

Front view

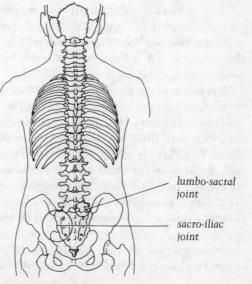

lumbo-sacral joint

sacro-iliac joint

Rear view

room for delivery of the baby's head.) These curves make for an increase in mechanical strength of the column.

The shape of the spine, though assumed by many to be constant, changes over time from the basic C-shape of the newborn infant to the elongated S-shape of puberty and adult life, before gradually reverting towards a modified C-shape in old age. The wedged shape of the bones in the region of the chest and pelvis contributes to these curves. In the neck and loin the curves are due primarily to the shape of the discs, and are maintained by the tension of muscles and ligaments.

Up to 25 per cent of the total length of the spinal column is made up by discs, and when the discs are removed from a spinal column and the bony components brought together, the spine forms into the C-shape as at birth. As the body ages, the intervertebral discs lose some of their height by a complicated process of chemical dehydration. In addition, even the bones may alter their shape through wear and tear and different chemical changes. This helps to explain why old people tend actually to shrink physically and to become bowed.

There are other components of the spinal column, which play a supporting and controlling role – namely the muscles and ligaments, without which we would not be able to function. These will be considered after we have made a more detailed examination of the relationship between the discs and the vertebrae, and of the important small joints at the back of the vertebrae.

Although there are many similarities between the vertebrae and discs at all levels of the spine, each one of these structures is uniquely designed to play its particular role in the function and action of the spinal column as a whole. As this book is concerned chiefly with the problems of the lower portion of the spine, the features of two lumbar vertebrae and their shared disc will be examined in greater depth.

Looking at the vertebrae from the front, there is a squat cylindrical area, a little like a flattened cotton reel, called the body, which has a hard outer layer and a honeycombed core. The bodies of adjacent vertebrae are separated by an intervertebral disc, which is fused to the surface of the vertebrae. At the rear of the vertebral body two columns of bone join together to form a tunnel which extends down the whole length of the spinal column to the junction of the fifth lumbar vertebra and the sacrum. This tunnel houses and protects the spinal cord to the level of the second lumbar vertebra, and a bundle of spinal nerves below this.

Exploded side view of vertebral segment

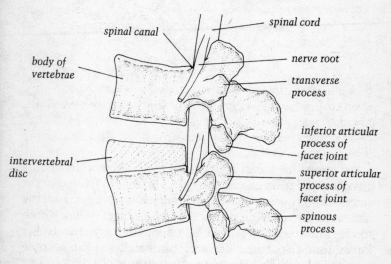

In addition, the arch which forms the spinal canal gives rise to some bony projections, the spinous processes – which you can feel if you run your fingers down the middle of your back – and also the transverse processes. These projections provide attachment for the muscles and ligaments of the spine, as well as helping to support the ribs. One other set of structures in this area is the facet joints, which link the vertebrae together at the rear. In addition they control and limit the range of movement between each pair of vertebrae. The intervertebral discs tend to lift and separate the vertebrae, facilitating freer movement between the various segments. The height of the discs determines the range, and the shape of the facet joints the direction, of possible movement.

Third lumbar vertebra viewed from above

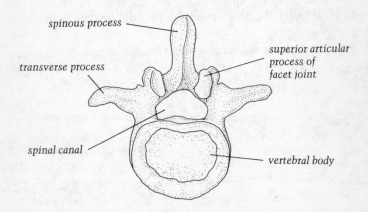

spinous process

superior articular process of facet joint

transverse process

spinal canal

vertebral body

As mentioned earlier, the spine is subject to ageing changes, and to an extent the rate of change is related to the stress that the structures are obliged to accept and the fitness of the individual concerned. The facet joints, which have similar capsules and ligaments to, say, the finger joints, tend to become less well lubricated and can become roughened, which obviously affects their efficiency. The intervertebral disc undergoes a more complicated chemical and mechanical process of change.

There are three components which make up a disc: the pads of cartilage which bond with the vertebrae above and below, the central jelly-like nucleus, and a surrounding 'corset' consisting of layers of crossply fibres. The central nucleus comes under pressure whenever we stand or sit up, and this pressure increases when carrying or lifting any weight. In about 15 per cent of the population who experience back pain, degenerative changes in the nucleus and outer ring of fibres, combined with wear and tear, may result in damage to the disc. Since the spinal cord and nerve roots lie in close proximity to the back of the disc, any change in shape to the disc, or any material that escapes from it, can press on a nerve root or even the spinal cord and produce severe pain and disability.

Areas of the Spine and Their Problems

The Neck

Known as the cervical spine, this area is made up of seven small and fairly delicate vertebrae. The first two – the atlas and axis – take the weight of the head on the neck. They also permit the head and upper spine to rotate without compromising the spinal cord and nerves. In total the head can rotate through a 180° arc. Half of this rotation occurs between the atlas and the axis, the remainder being produced between the other five vertebrae. Further, the shape of the facet joints allows the head to be bent forwards, backwards and to both sides.

The combination of repeated and free movement and the considerable weight of the head, which has to be supported by the cervical spine, makes the vertebrae and discs prone to wear and tear. This occurs most often in the fifth, sixth and seventh vertebrae. Actual ruptures of the cervical discs are relatively rare, compared to the lumbar region, although sudden traction force on the arms or a whiplash injury of the sort that may be experienced in road traffic accidents may precipitate a true disc problem.

Should the cervical spine become worn, there may be changes to the normal range of movements between the various component parts as well as some narrowing of the spaces through which the nerve roots pass. This can result in nerves' being nipped or even trapped. The pain which is produced is usually felt in the neck, shoulder, elbow and fingers, and the condition is called cervical spondylosis. Physiotherapists, who are regularly asked to treat 'tennis elbows', always have to make sure that this is an accurate diagnosis and that the pain has not been referred from undetected damage in the neck.

Very severe pain may require rest in bed, but usually treatment involves wearing a cervical collar or gentle manipulation. Most incidences of cervical spondylosis resolve in a matter of weeks. It should be noted, however, that whilst a collar provides some support for the neck it is important to avoid rotation of the head and neck until the symptoms have subsided.

The Chest
The thoracic spine is the longest segment in the spinal column, and is made up of twelve vertebrae. A pair of ribs is attached to each vertebra by means of additional specialized joints. Movements in this part of the spine, with the exception of rotation, are restricted, thus providing the stability needed by the heart, lungs, and other organs contained within the rib cage.

Injuries to the thoracic spine are fairly rare, though road accidents or a heavy fall on to the upper back may result in a crush fracture of a vertebral body. Sometimes people complain of a local ache at a particular level in their chest, which feels as if there is a tight string tied round it. This means pressure on a nerve, and whilst it is frequently due to some minor damage it is important before seeking physiotherapy to exclude more serious trouble. You should visit your doctor and an X-ray may be required.

The Lower Back
An exploratory feel round your own lumbar spine will reveal that the vertebrae in this region are larger and more ruggedly constructed than the vertebrae in the neck and chest region. The discs are also thicker and more substantially developed. The lumbar spine takes the weight of the head, neck, trunk, arms, and anything that is carried, and transmits the load to the pelvis and legs. Additionally, up to 70 per cent of the bending in the lower spine takes place in the third, fourth and fifth lumbar vertebral segments and the junction between the fifth lumbar vertebra and the top

of the sacrum. Not surprisingly this area suffers the highest incidence of wear and tear, some of which could be avoided by learning simple techniques of lifting. About 85 per cent of cases of rupture of the fibres or prolapse of the central nucleus of the disc occur in this region.

Research indicates that anyone over the age of fifty is almost certain to have degenerative changes in the fifth lumbar disc and to a lesser degree in the third and fourth lumbar discs as well.

The Sacral Segment

Although damage to the sacrum can be caused by direct trauma like a car crash, it is otherwise fairly rare for pain to arise in this region. Most problems result either from strain and irritation of the lumbo-sacral joint, which is the junction between the spine and the pelvis, or from the sacro-iliac joints between the sacrum and the two hip bones. The latter become more lax in pregnancy, but argument still rages as to whether or not there is movement at other times.

The Coccyx

Injury to the coccyx, man's residual tail, can be the cause of back pain which is localized to the buttocks and between the thighs. Direct injury, such as a heavy fall on the base of the spine, is the most common cause of the pain called coccydynia. This nasty, literally deep-seated pain is not always easy to treat, and is aggravated by sitting and going to the toilet.

Supporting Structures

The vertebrae are linked by ligaments, strong fibrous bands of various lengths, as well as by discs and the joints at the back of the spinal canal. The spinal column is further supported by the muscles of the back and abdomen. Holding a deep breath raises pressure in the chest and abdomen, always assuming the muscles of the pelvic floor are in good order, and this provides additional bracing for the spine.

The Ligaments

The functions of the ligaments and the joint capsules of the spinal column are to provide stability to the structure, to control and guide movement, and to prevent damage from too much motion in the various segments. The significance of spinal ligaments is only now beginning to be appreciated, and when damaged they may play an important part in the production of pain.

The spinal ligaments

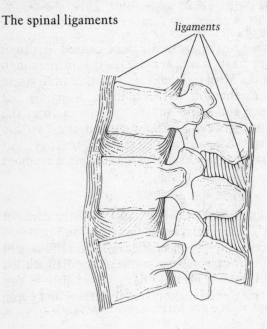

ligaments

With the exception of the yellow elastic ligaments of the spine, the remainder can be compared to the cables used to support large aerial masts. Their chief function is to take the loading and tension applied to the spine, and because they are passive structures the tension developed within them is related directly to their length and cross-section. The strength of the ligament when it is under loading will depend on its size and shape and on the speed at which the load is applied.

When stressed under normal circumstances, without any excessive loading and at a reasonable rate, the ligaments are able to accept the strain applied. If they are loaded very quickly, subjected to sustained pressure or exposed to repeated stress, the fibres can become stretched and deformed and may even tear. This may then produce instability and have a knock-on effect on other structures.

Ligaments respond to the mechanical demands placed on them by becoming stronger and stiffer. Thus the person who is regularly working on a heavy task involving the spine is protected to a certain extent by beneficial adaptive changes in the body. It is worth noting that the muscles provide the first line of defence for the spinal column and the ligaments provide a back-up system. Lack of stimulation from exercise can lead to weakened muscles and ligaments which may lose their tensile load-bearing ability, making them more readily damaged by sudden unexpected activity. There would seem to be some very good arguments, therefore, for limiting bed-rest to as long only as it takes for inflammation and pain to settle down.

It is a common belief that a feeling of fatigue in the joints, particularly in the spine, is due to muscle tiredness, but it is much more likely that this sensation is caused by tension and strain on the ligaments and joint capsules. Sitting with a poor posture tends to place significant strain on the ligaments of the spine and probably accounts for much of the low-grade backache that occurs in sedentary workers, in drivers of cars and heavy lorries, and in schoolchildren.

The Spinal Muscles

These may be considered in three broad groups – the muscles at the back, at the sides and at the front of the spine. All spinal muscles, in addition to producing motion, also serve to maintain the stability of the trunk and to counteract the effects of gravity. When the spine bends forwards there is a gradual increase in activity in the large spinal muscles in the lumbar region. (However, when the spine approaches the final few degrees of forward bend these muscles cease to function, possibly because they are no longer necessary as the ligaments, particularly the yellow elastic ligaments, are on full stretch and accepting the load. The stress placed on the ligaments is very high and may, on occasions, exceed their maximum loading levels and cause some form of damage.) When the trunk is raised from the stooped position, the spinal muscles begin to work after the first few degrees of straightening (there

The spinal muscles

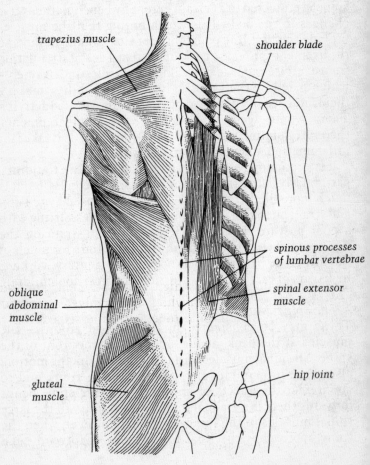

seems to be a particular 'on-off' point). Initially they work very strongly, gradually reducing their activity as the normal erect position is achieved and the effects of leverage are reduced.

The implications of this, when it comes to stoop-lifting, are fairly obvious. Fatigue in the back muscles is directly proportionate to the loading applied and the length of time during which activity takes place. There is a real need for frequent rest periods or change of activity when undertaking heavy work, particularly if it is not part of your normal routine. Fatigue can have cumulative effects which may not appear for some hours afterwards. A number of back pain sufferers who reported that they woke up with their pain revealed that they had been working in the garden or moving house a day or so before. The old admonition to 'put your back into it' is really not a good idea.

The Abdominal Muscles

Although these may be involved to an extent in sideways bending and rotation of the trunk, their particular role is associated with the increase of pressure in the abdominal cavity. This pressure, which develops naturally and automatically whenever we lift objects, especially in the initial stages, helps to counteract and reduce the mechanical loading on the spine. The reduction of spinal stress resulting from intra-abdominal pressure in the 'working male or female' can be as high as 25 per cent, but the housewife or office worker who is not involved in regular lifting and whose muscular tone may be less specifically developed can often only achieve a 13 per cent reduction in spinal loading. As helpful as intra-abdominal pressure is, when it is sustained over a long period – particularly when associated with a heavy load – it can lead to hernias in both sexes and, on occasion, to uterine prolapse in women with poor tone or tear damage after childbirth. The importance of good pelvic floor and abdominal muscle tone for women cannot be overstressed. It is especially important that antenatal and postnatal exercises are properly supervised and encouraged.

The Spinal Cord

The spinal cord is connected to the brain at the base of the skull and continues down the spine, within the spinal canal, to the upper border of the second lumbar vertebra, below which point the nerve roots divide to supply the lower limbs. At each vertebral junction there are a pair of nerves, one on either side, which emerge through a space called the intervertebral foramen. The cord and nerve roots

The spinal cord

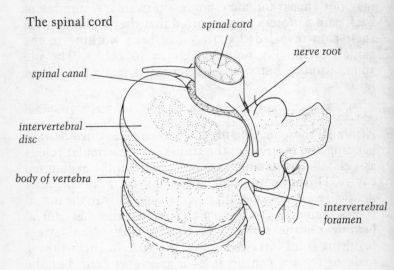

are covered by a sleeve of protective membranes containing cerebrospinal fluid, which permits free movement of the spinal cord within the spinal canal as well as acting as a shock-absorbing buffer.

If we consider the brain as a specialized controlling mechanism like a highly complex computerized telephone network, then the spinal cord is the trunking which permits the rapid transmission of messages to and from the various parts of the body. Much of the body's functioning is automatic, and directly under the control of the master programme. This then permits us to concentrate on and think about the specific needs of a given moment, and saves us from an overload of information.

The spinal cord is located directly behind the body of the vertebrae when viewed from the front. In cross-section the spinal canal is roughly circular, though it varies in the individual segments. Recent research has shown that some people, whose spinal canal is reduced in size as a part of their normal make-up, are more vulnerable to back pain caused by spinal cord and nerve root compression. This is because the space around the cord is very limited and even minor changes in overall spinal relationships can produce pain. Because of the close relationship between the disc, spinal cord, nerve roots and vertebrae, it is not too difficult to imagine how the nerve roots can become compressed and/or tethered by alterations in the shape of the discs or of the vertebrae themselves, due to wear and tear.

If the spinal cord were not housed within the spinal column, then injury to the spine would be no more serious than similar injuries to other bones and joints. When it is realized as well that at least nine separate types of structures related to the spine can produce pain, it may be easier to understand some of the reasons why back pain is so difficult to diagnose and to treat.

Nerve root compression

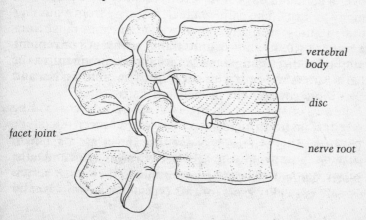

vertebral body

disc

facet joint

nerve root

2 *Common Types and Causes of Back Pain*

Because back pain is such a complex syndrome it is difficult to give anything other than a broad outline of its more common causes. Whilst, therefore, it is comforting to have some idea of what has gone wrong, it is best to approach any attempts at self-diagnosis with great caution.

Although Chapter 3 will provide you with some simple ways of easing your discomfort, it is important to learn how to differentiate between a minor injury which will respond to home treatment and the more serious type requiring professional medical attention. As a general rule, if you have very severe pain or significant discomfort which persists for more than twenty-four hours, then you should see your doctor. Watch out for deep-seated pain radiating from the lower back, particularly if going down one or both legs and possibly accompanied by pins and needles, numbness or extra sensitivity to touch. Such symptoms must never be ignored and require prompt attention.

Back pain may be sudden in onset or develop gradually over a period of days. It may resolve quickly or persist for many months. The pain you feel may arise from a number of structures within the spinal system, and may range from a minor ache to almost unbearable agony. A convenient method of discussing some of the more common origins of back pain is to begin with the superficial soft tissues and then work towards the deeper spinal structures.

Soft Tissue Injuries

These develop as a result of over-use and strain, or sudden changes in position as experienced in slips, trips and falls. Sports, gardening, house-moving and do-it-yourself activities are typical triggers for this type of back pain. Usually those who keep themselves fit and active are less likely to suffer such an injury, although anyone may lay themselves open to damage through sudden and unexpected movements, especially when the body is already pre-stressed by poor posture and/or cumulative fatigue. The main structures involved are the muscles and ligaments.

Muscle Strains

Strains or tears are normally fairly minor in nature and can begin with a sharp pain, which gradually fades to a dull ache and local tenderness. The most likely cause is that some muscle fibres and the connective tissues containing the muscle bundles have become over-stretched or even torn. There may be some associated swelling and minor bleeding and bruising. Those who are young and fit will be able to work off the after-effects of injury in a few days. In the older or less fit individual recovery is likely to take longer, particularly if there has been previous damage.

Sometimes people experience pain in the superficial spinal muscles, often in the neck and shoulder region, without any obvious history of injury. The term 'fibrositis' is frequently used, although no one has been able to demonstrate any changes in the structures involved, other than muscle tenderness and spasm. With this condition, it is possible to demonstrate so-called 'trigger-spots'. Pressing these spots exaggerates the pain, and injection of local anaesthetic or gentle massage may relieve it. The most predictable causes of 'fibrositis' are poor posture, tension or exposure to cold and draughts.

Ligamentous Injuries

These are caused by overstretching or tearing the fibres. Ligaments are tough but if torn heal slowly and poorly, unlike muscles which have a much better blood supply. The majority of acute injuries to ligaments occur from sudden unexpected bending or twisting applied to an unguarded spine. Because the forces developed are large, it is not uncommon for muscles to be torn as well. A tendency to exceed normal ranges of movement is guarded against by an automatic contraction of muscles which produce the opposite effect. Signals to these protecting muscles come from joint capsules as well as from stretched muscles. If the system is caught unawares this useful safeguard does not operate and tissues may be damaged.

A slower form of ligamentous damage may be produced by repeated low-level stress in the form of poor standing or sitting positions. Stop for a moment and check how you are sitting or standing. It is almost certain that your lower back will be rounded abnormally, either in a forward or backward position. When this position remains unsupported for more than a few minutes, the ligaments stretch and deform. This loss of tensile strength is not easy to restore. There can also be a knock-on effect upon the spinal segments, with instability and degenerative changes possibly occurring as a result. Alternatively, a worn disc could alter the way in which a vertebra relates to those above and below it, placing constant low-grade abnormal strain on the ligaments and other soft structures.

Ligamentous tears may be microscopic, or may extend across the whole ligament. If an injury to a ligament is caused by sudden force, there will be acute pain, followed by swelling and protective muscle spasm. With rest, the symptoms settle to a more deep-seated ache, which may flare into acute pain on sudden early movement before healing is complete. Chronic strains develop more slowly and are felt as aches and 'tiredness'. As the condition progresses, the ache settles into an ever-present gnawing and even grinding pain. If posture is poor, healing will only be speeded up if corrective measures are taken.

Similar types of aches or pains occur when tears develop in points of attachment of soft tissues into bone other than the spine, for example the rim of the pelvis or around the hip and groin. Even small tears of this nature can produce a lot of pain over a wide area. Because there is a natural tendency to blame all pain in the lower trunk and limbs on the spine, this sort of injury may be misdiagnosed and confused with more serious damage.

Spinal Injuries

Fractures of the Spine

Unless associated with secondary disease or with the chemical and physical changes in bone which are called osteoporosis, direct trauma is the chief cause of fractures of the spine. A fall, car crash, or a direct blow to the spine can all lead to a crack in the transverse or spinous processes at the back of the vertebrae or to a crushing deformity of the vertebral body. The exact force required to produce such an injury will vary with the circumstances and the age of the individual. In the elderly, a sudden unguarded step off a pavement edge could be sufficient to produce a crack fracture in one of the vertebrae. How much pain results seems to bear no relationship to the severity of the injury. Fractures of the transverse processes can sometimes be very painful, as can some crush fractures of the vertebral bodies in the thoracic spine. On the other hand, there are many people who never discover that they have sustained any injury at all until they have a routine X-ray for some other investigation.

Injuries to Facet Joints

Like most other small joints, these have an enclosing capsule, ligaments and a very rich nerve supply. There are good reasons to believe that more instances of back pain

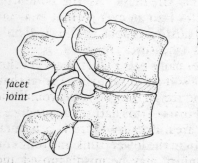

Joint separation

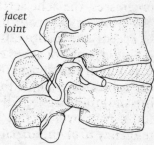

Nerve root entrapment

are occasioned as a result of injury to or disturbance of these joints than had until recently been thought. Strains to the facet joints are normally produced by bending and twisting actions which separate the joints beyond their normal range. If the force and movement are great enough the joint can become misaligned. Surprisingly, the pain which accompanies this event can be very intense and diffuse in its distribution. In consequence of this, and because of the muscle spasm which also occurs, patients and those who treat them cannot be blamed for thinking a disc injury is present, as the pain patterns experienced by those with facet joint injuries at a particular level mimic those which follow a disc injury at the same level. It is sometimes difficult to reach a correct diagnosis and patients can become increasingly frustrated as no one seems able to find the true cause of their pain. With the ever-growing popularity of the manipulative techniques, prompt diagnosis combined with appropriate treatment can resolve many facet joint problems in a relatively short time. However, it is important to seek advice at an early stage if treatment is to be successful.

Sacro-Iliac Strains

The sacro-iliac joint, where the sacrum and two hip bones meet, is a common site of pain. There are two main schools

The pelvis

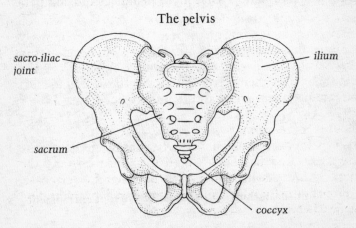

sacro-iliac joint

ilium

sacrum

coccyx

of thought amongst practitioners. One group, though it accepts that there is some joint laxity during pregnancy, questions whether or not there is movement at other times and believes that pain in this area is referred from other structures within the spinal system. The remainder are convinced that there is some movement in the sacro-iliac joints, particularly but not only in women whose ligaments are slackened by hormonal activity during pregnancy and menstruation. The latter viewpoint would apear to be the more likely.

Sacro-iliac strains are normally caused by bending and twisting movements of the spine, when the legs are firmly fixed. The sacro-iliac joint on the opposite side to the one of bend or twist may be subjected to large turning forces, and this may cause some slight but significant displacement between the joint surfaces. If this is not corrected there may be associated effects on the spinal column above it, producing a spiralling pattern of pain and, if severe enough, muscle spasm.

An uncomplicated sacro-iliac strain will begin with pain over the joint line. This pain may radiate into the groin on the same side. If there are reflected disturbances to the spinal column above, there could be pain in one or more sites higher up. With an injury of the right sacro-iliac joint the typical pattern would be pain in the right sacro-iliac joint, then in the lower or mid-lumbar spine on the left and the lower thoracic spine on the right. As in other regions of the spine, persistent strains of this joint can develop into more permanent degenerative changes, not only in the sacro-iliac joints themselves but also in the discs and facet joints immediately above in the lumbo-sacral area.

Acute Disc Lesions

This type of back problem was first identified during the early 1930s and has been called a 'slipped disc' by the general public. As discs do not slip between the vertebrae, the proper term for a disc injury is a prolapsed intervertebral disc or P.I.D.

Like any other structure, this specialized pad of shock-absorbing tissue undergoes changes as a result of the ageing process. The rate of change will be accelerated in those discs subject to the most stress, primarily in the lower lumbar region. Two components of the disc are chiefly involved – the outer layers of crossply fibres, called the annulus, and the central pulpy nucleus. Often changes occur in both structures at the same time. Simple degeneration of the nucleus is due to both chemical changes in its structure and a gradual invasion by fibres from the annulus. The nucleus, which in the healthy disc resembles cellulose wallpaper paste, changes over time to a porridge-like consistency, and later comes to resemble the stringy texture of white crabmeat. Ultimately the disc may become a solid mass of tissue which can, in some instances, wear away.

In conjunction with these age-related changes, repeated minor stress or more severe loading of the spine in a bent or twisted posture may cause the layers of the annulus to shear apart, forming small cracks. Gradually these cracks develop into larger fissures through which the nucleus may eventually rupture. The material which bursts out, like an egg cracking in boiling water, goes backwards into the vertebral canal and presses on the nerve root or even the spinal cord, causing the severe pain that people wrongly attribute to a 'slipped disc'.

Those who experience a prolapse of the intervertebral disc are likely to be between the ages of twenty-five and fifty years. In the under twenty-fives the discs are well able to resist the forces which are applied to them, whilst in the over-fifties the discs have reached a stage where prolapse is unlikely to occur because of the ageing changes that have taken place. The popular image of an acute disc attack is of someone lifting a heavy object using a bent back and straight leg lift. Suddenly they collapse with a cry, holding their lower back. In a state of shock the victim staggers to some convenient couch and waits for medical attention, before being helped into bed.

Disc rupture (top view)

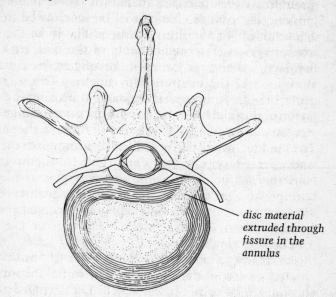

disc material
extruded through
fissure in the
annulus

Disc rupture (side view)

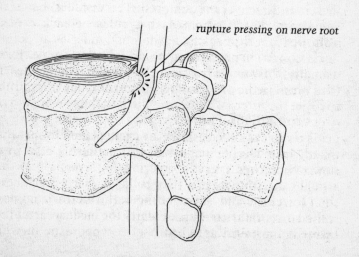

rupture pressing on nerve root

In reality this is the exception rather than the rule. The prelude to an attack is frequently a period of heavy prolonged activity such as gardening, moving house or the adoption of poor working postures. The individual often complains of being tired or having a sore, stiff back. Some hours or even days later, whilst undertaking a simple activity, like sitting up in bed, coughing, or going to the toilet, the person experiences a sensation like a minor explosion in the lower part of the back. Depending on the severity and the location of the disc rupture, there will be pain in the lower back, possibly spreading down the leg on the affected side. Movement may be difficult and the sufferer will bend the spine to the opposite side in an attempt to ease the pressure on the trapped nerve roots. The main symptoms are invariably accompanied by muscle spasm, which leads to the 'spasm – pain – spasm' cycle. This can be very troublesome.

For many, a short period of bed rest, warmth and analgesics settles the condition. The initial inflammation subsides and the disc reseals itself. The extruded material shrinks and over a period of weeks is eventually dissolved by the body. Gradually the sufferer is able to resume normal activities, though it may take up to three months before full recovery is achieved. The disc will have been weakened, but if commonsense rules of back care are followed and the back and abdominal muscles are kept in good condition there need be no further trouble. Exceptionally, this simple treatment may fail to relieve the pain, and orthopaedic or neurological surgery may be required.

Chronic Back Pain

This term is used to describe a variety of conditions which result in low-grade, persistent or fluctuating pain in the lower back over a very long period.

The causative factors may be degenerative changes in the vertebrae and surrounding soft tissues, commonly called osteoarthritis. In the elderly the basic wear and tear may be increased as a result of osteoporosis, in which metabolic changes in the bone make it more porous and liable to collapse, and the problem is added to by the gradual changes in the discs.

Another common cause of chronic back pain is increased movement between segments of the spine due to a combination of changes in the discs, ligaments and muscles working on the joints at the back of the spinal segment. Any forces which are placed on these unstable or misaligned spinal segments will not be distributed in an even manner, as they would be in a healthy and normal stable spine. As a result the already weakened and damaged structures are placed under added stress causing swelling, inflammation and pain. Activities such as sitting in a poor position, standing for long periods, and unaccustomed work involving bending and lifting will result in an increase of pain and discomfort in the lower back.

Persistent pain in the lower spinal region may also be caused if the nerve roots are squeezed within a narrowed spinal canal. Similarly, the space through which the nerve root passes may be restricted by bony outgrowths on the facet joints. Both these conditions may on occasions be improved by surgery.

A small percentage of the population has a congenital mechanical weakness of the spinal arch, usually at either the lumbo-sacral joint or between the fourth and fifth lumbar vertebrae. This is called spondylosis. In some instances one of the vertebrae may shear and the condition becomes known as spondylolisthesis. Occasionally surgical measures may be required to stabilize the spine at the affected level. If you are told that you have one of these conditions you might like to ask to look at your X-rays. It may be possible to show you exactly what is wrong.

Gynaecological Backache

After dysmenorrhea, the most common occasion for gynaecological back pain is during and after pregnancy. The gradual weight increase and shift of centre of gravity alters the balance of the body and there is an exaggeration of the lumbar curve, giving rise in the latter stages to the familiar 'I am proud to be pregnant' posture. As a result of the changes in weight distribution, the ligaments and muscles which support the spine are placed under increasing stress and the problem is made even worse as the ligaments slacken in response to hormonal changes.

Unless the backache is identified at an early stage and corrective measures taken, it is possible for the pain to continue for months after the baby is born. Supervised instruction on proper posture, the provision of a suitable spinal support, and ante- and postnatal exercises can all help to resolve this type of back pain.

Although a number of gynaecological conditions may aggravate pre-existing backache, it is highly unlikely that most gynaecological complaints would initiate back pain on their own. If your back pain appears to be linked to periods, sexual intercourse or other general dragging pelvic aches, it is best to seek the advice of your doctor in order to eliminate these gynaecological factors and to assist in the resolution of the whole problem.

Inflammatory Back Pain

About 4 per cent of those who experience back pain do not exhibit symptoms commonly associated with a mechanical disorder. It is easy to dismiss the patient as someone whose problem is purely in the mind, but this could mean that a very real condition is overlooked.

One of the best known of inflammatory conditions is ankylosing spondylitis, in which the joints of the spine become inflamed and there is a gradual change in the ligaments and capsules which are converted into bone. This complaint is far more common in men than women. It requires blood tests and X-ray examinations before a firm diagnosis can be made, and if you are told that you have ankylosing spondylitis your specialist should provide you with all the necessary support, advice and treatment that you require.

Outside the diagnosis of ankylosing spondylitis there are

several lesser inflammatory conditions which require careful assessment by a consultant specializing in rheumatology. The symptoms of inflammatory conditions of the spine tend to extend over a number of spinal segments and can be fleeting in nature. Pain is normally worse on lying down and after periods of inactivity. Activity and gentle exercise appear to ease the pain. Quite frequently there is no history of injury to the back and the patient may complain of feeling off-colour.

As inflammatory back pain is due to chemical irritation in the spinal joints, physical measures do not provide lasting relief, although heat may ease the local tenderness for a while. Some form of anti-inflammatory drug therapy is required and normally, once a clear diagnosis has been made and a suitable treatment begun, the results are very good.

Understanding Your Reaction to Back Pain

Have you ever wondered why back pain seems to produce such dramatic symptoms when a person with crippling arthritis is apparently able to cope with their pain and disability?

Pain, particularly when the problem reaches a chronic state, is not a purely physical complaint but is overlaid with varying degrees of psychological response as well. Modern theories of pain suggest that it is an unpleasant emotional disorder due to stimulation of special receptors in the tissues, which signal that something is amiss. The trigger factor may be mechanical or chemical in nature. If the signal initiated is of sufficient intensity the message is passed up to the pain centres in the brain, by means of the special tracts in the spinal cord. Once the signal arrives at the pain centres, links are established with other areas of the brain and the original input is modified by past experience, current mental and physical states and the significance of the pain at that time. So when the pain finally registers at a conscious level the primary signal may have been appreciably modified.

One explanation of why damage to the spinal region initiates an enhanced response is that the back is involved in so many of our daily activities, such as lying down, sitting, standing and walking. Also, if there is nerve root entrapment, sneezing, coughing, and all forms of straining can increase the pain. Thus the pain is not only the central focal point and ever-present, but is intensified as well by a variety of simple repetitive normal activities.

Those who have never experienced such pain for themselves find it all too easy to think that all back pain sufferers are lead-swingers or, at least, that many of their problems are imagined. The unfortunate result is that people tend to treat back pain in others as a joke. It is dangerous to dismiss any claim of back pain on the grounds of malingering, without a full and detailed examination of all the facts.

CHANCES OF RECOVERY		
Minor episode	—	Very good
Soft tissue injury	—	Good
Facet joint injury	—	Good to fair
Repeated episodic back pain and disc involvement	—	Poor to fair depending on severity of damage and treatment adpoted

Very few back pain sufferers cannot be helped to achieve a more normal lifestyle, provided they are given the proper treatment and advice, and have a positive attitude towards the resolution of their complaint.

In an exceedingly small number of cases back pain may be used for the purposes of malingering. Also, there are instances where people may tend to exaggerate and prolong their symptoms for some form of gain at an unconscious level, but the pain and symptoms are nevertheless real to most of them, and careful treatment and guidance is therefore still required if the matter is to be resolved. The malingerer, on the other hand, uses back pain as an excuse, or to achieve some particular conscious aim. Usually this can be detected at an early stage of the medical investigation, but regrettably such cases, few as they are, perpetuate a false attitude to genuine back pain.

The most important part of any treatment for back pain is to try to gain an understanding of the cause and significance of the symptoms. When attempting to evaluate your pain for yourself, or when describing it to your doctor, it is essential to be as objective as possible, and to note carefully the location of the pain and the factors that relieve or accentuate it, in order to assist in arriving at a diagnosis.

3 *Self-Help and Self-Assessment*

The chapter which follows should help you to cope with minor episodes of back pain and suggest ways of easing an acute attack until you can obtain professional medical assistance. Much of the advice is based on simple tried remedies and common sense.

How Bad Is It?

Before contemplating any form of self-treatment, it is vitally important that you are able to recognize the difference between a fairly minor episode and the more serious event which requires the expert attention of your doctor or health adviser. The self-assessment form which follows should provide an aid to identifying the site and distribution of your pain and the other symptoms that may be present. It is not intended to lead to an actual diagnosis, but rather to let you examine your symptoms in an objective and logical manner. This will not only help you but will also be useful for your doctor, should medical attention be necessary.

Read the questions carefully all the way through, before attempting to complete the questionnaire. You may want to make a few rough notes as you go along. Try to answer the questions as honestly and logically as possible; really think about what you are putting down. If this is done properly you should end up with a reasonable idea of exactly where your pain is, even though you may not appreciate its source. When your pain seems to be limited to the muscles and soft structures and there is no central spinal pain, it is likely that you have strained yourself. If the pain is severe and there is deep-seated pain in and around the spine, possibly going down into the legs, *this needs checking with your doctor without delay*. If the pain is such that movement is difficult, rest is the best immediate solution, whilst you wait for your doctor to call.

SELF-ASSESSMENT QUESTIONNAIRE

---

1. *Brief History*

When did your pain begin (time and date)?

How did it start – suddenly or gradually?

Was there anything that brought it on, e.g. lifting, twisting, sneezing?

Had you undertaken any abnormal activity over the previous few days before your attack?

Have you had back pain before?

If so, how many times, and when?

Was it as bad as your present attack?

What eases your pain?

What aggravates your pain?

2. *Site of Your Pain*

On the diagram overleaf, show where you can feel the pain. If there is a particularly painful area mark it with a *, as accurately as you can.

If the pain spreads from one area to another, use a line of arrows to show its path (see example).

Should you experience numbness or pins and needles, mark the area with ▦ for pins and needles and ▨ for numbness.

3. *Severity of Pain*

It is useful to try to evaluate the severity of the pain you are experiencing. In order to have some form of comparison think of the worst pain you have ever had. This will be the highest level. Try to be as accurate as possible

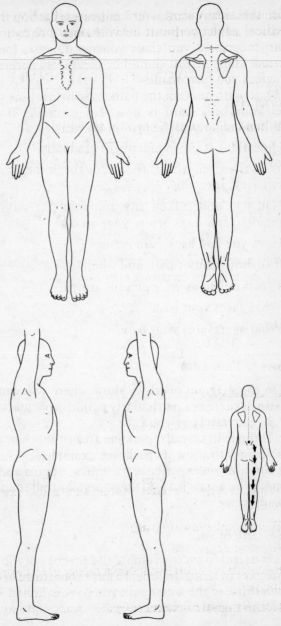

with this, as any score over 7 indicates that you should seek medical advice without delay. It may help you to check your progress if you chart your pain over a fourteen-day period. Many of you should be pleasantly surprised at the progress you have made.

Mark with an X on the pain scale below how severe you feel your back pain is now. For example, if you have minimal pain it will be low on the scale:

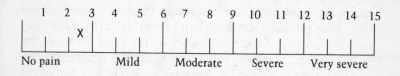

If you have very severe pain you will be unable to rest, sleep, or think of anything else.

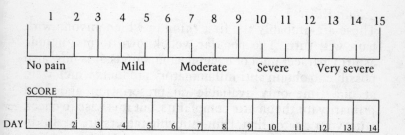

4. *General Health*

What is your present state of physical and mental health?

Have you been run down?

Are you depressed?

If so, did this depression begin before or after the onset of the pain?

Has the depression increased?

Easing Mild Back Pain

Although the pain from any form of back injury can feel really dreadful, it usually diminishes in a few hours, particularly after rest. However impossible it may sound, try to relax. Apprehension is understandable, but the majority of episodes are resolved in less than a month, and most attacks settle down in a few days. Fear and pain only help to increase muscle tension, so adding to the overall discomfort. Since muscle spasm is one of the most common factors in back pain, any reduction of this tension should therefore produce some real and tangible relief. Don't get too despondent if the pain returns after a few hours at the outset, as the period of relief will gradually lengthen.

As well as relaxation and exercise, which will be discussed later, some of the simple and well tried short-term remedies which you may find helpful – even if you also decide to consult your doctor – include pain-relieving tablets, hot and cold therapy, vibration and massage.

Pain Killers

These are probably the first thing to which anyone with pain will turn. The popular well known forms include aspirin, paracetamol or codeine compounds. It is now also possible to obtain anti-inflammatory products which were at one time only available on prescription and used primarily for rheumatic complaints, but it is wise to check with your doctor first. Pain-relieving tablets are useful in the early stages to control acute pain and reduce spasm, although by themselves they do not promote healing. They should not be taken on an empty stomach, and in some instances there could be unpleasant side-effects such as heartburn, nausea or constipation. Probably the best way to use this kind of relief is at bedtime, as an aid to getting some sound sleep.

The Use of Heat and Cold

When back pain is due to muscular or ligamentous strain, it is possible that there may be some associated bruising. During the first forty-eight hours, any form of heat other than the gentlest warmth will tend to increase the local circulation. This aggravates the swelling and spasm, and initially therefore cold therapy will probably be more effective. An alternative is to use arnica ointment, which can have an almost miraculous effect when applied to bruised and tender areas. Once the injury has had a chance to settle down, heat may be more beneficial, as an increase in the local circulation at this stage is desirable and promotes healing of torn tissues. *Never use heat or ice over any area where sensation is diminished or not present.*

Cold Therapy

Cold therapy is most easily applied by means either of cold towels or of cold packs. For the former you will need four small handtowels and a medium-sized bowl, which is used to hold a mixture of crushed ice and water. Once you have made the ice and water mix into a thin slush, put the four towels into the bowl to soak while you uncover the part you want to treat and settle down into a suitable and comfortable position. Take one or two towels out of the bowl and wring them almost dry before applying them in a pad to your back. Leave them in position for two minutes before changing the towels for those still in the iced water. Repeat this procedure for 10–15 minutes in any one treatment. Up to three treatments a day are in order, as long as you leave around two hours between each session to give time for the treatment to have an effect and for the circulation to return to normal.

A more convenient method of applying cold is with cold packs. Ideally, use a flexible ice pack sold for use in cold boxes and freezer shopping bags. Another good alternative is to fill a rubber hot-water bottle with crushed ice and water to make an ice bag. If neither of these is available you could use ice and water sealed in a strong polythene bag, or even an 8 oz pack of frozen peas. (Remember either to eat the peas once they have thawed or mark the packet clearly 'not to be eaten' if you wish to re-freeze the peas for use again!)

Because it is fairly easy to suffer an ice burn, always wrap the ice pack in a just-damp terry towel which has been soaked in cold water. *Before applying the pack use a piece of tissue or cotton wool to wipe the area to be treated with olive oil or vegetable oil. Never apply any form of ice directly on to the skin.* Once you have put the pack into position, cover it with a layer of polythene and use a crepe bandage to bind it into place. Limit your first treatment to 10 minutes and as long as you have no adverse effects increase the treatment by 5 minutes each time, up to a total of 25 minutes.

At the end of the treatment remove the cold pack, wipe off the oil and get someone to check the skin of the treated area for signs of local redness or irritation. If you have followed the instructions carefully, there should be no problems. *However, if your skin has reacted adversely to the cold, you should stop the treatment.*

Therapeutic Heat

For this, a heat lamp is ideal but an electrically heated pad, available at most leading chemists, or a covered hot-water bottle, are reasonable alternatives. Do not use fierce heat as this could result in a burn or at least a semi-permanent blotchy pigmentation. Never apply heat, either, to any part that has been rubbed with liniment – you may prefer your back pain to the result produced! When using warmth, limit each treatment to 20 minutes and always check the skin after treatment.

The choice of either heat or cold is yours, as both have similar end-results, provided you take into consideration the stage of pain. To repeat the general principle, cold therapy is useful to reduce swelling during the early period and heat therapy is probably more soothing and relaxing, and particularly suitable for use in the later stages of an attack.

Vibration

Vibration, in the form of a motorized pad, can be an aid to relaxation and help to ease back pain. Research has shown that a speed of 50 cycles per second is the most beneficial, when the vibration pad is used for around 30 minutes.

Massage

This form of treatment has been used for thousands of years right back to the ancient civilizations of China, India, Greece and Rome. The effects of massage relate directly to the type of technique employed, and in the case of back pain the aims should be to relieve pain, to aid relaxation and to increase the local circulation. If, however, you find that massage increases the pain, do not continue with it. It will not relieve pain due to inflammatory diseases.

As few people have a natural ability to massage effectively, only two simple techniques will be described here – massage using the whole hand for deep general stroking, and massage using the fingers for local kneading. (Should you wish, you could of course visit your local physiotherapist, who specializes in massage.)

Stroking massage. To massage your own back, you should be sitting on a stool or the edge of a bed. Massage should be done with relaxed hands, the palms of which are placed in contact with the area of the back which is painful. Place your hands level with the lowest ribs, with the fingertips of both resting lightly on the spine just touching each other. Push your hands down towards the hips in a slow, steady stroke, and allow them to follow the line of the hips. Take them off and start again, trying to establish a smooth rhythm. Remember that the secret is to let the hands mould to the underlying tissues and do not tense up. You can practise on your forearm first to gain the necessary relaxation of the hands.

Finger kneadings. These are ideal for treating local areas of tenderness which are no larger than three inches in diameter. The pads of two or three fingers are placed in contact with the skin and moved in a circular motion. Start lightly and then add a little more pressure each time, but avoid digging in. Move the fingers round slowly in order to cover the whole area.

It may help you to massage more effectively if you use a little hand cream or aromatic oil. A word of caution, however: a number of lotions and creams containing 'warming agents' like capsicum are available. Although these provide local warmth and can assist muscle relaxation *they should be used carefully*, as some may prove to be too fierce for sensitive skins. If you use any liniments or creams, always wash your hands thoroughly afterwards before doing anything else.

Acute and Severe Attacks – How to Survive Them

In the early stages of an acute episode of back pain you may find that movement of any sort aggravates your pain, and the natural and instinctive reaction is to tense up and remain immobile. How much rest will be needed will depend on the severity and cause of the problem. (If there is only mild discomfort after a few hours, then a regime of restricted activity in which you avoid bending, twisting and lifting for a few days should soon restore you to normal.) When there is every indication that the pain is of a more serious nature – and you will certainly know the difference – then:

1. Contact your doctor and arrange for a visit as soon as possible.
2. Whilst you are waiting for medical attention, rest in any position that eases the pain. Most experts advocate the use of a good mattress on a firm base, so if your bed has a poor base get help to place the mattress on the floor for a few days and, when you are better, think seriously about buying a new bed. The use of a board will firm up the base but as it is likely that, if the base is worn, the mattress will be worn too, a new bed is the ideal solution. There

are instances where a good bed has completely cured long-term back-ache. (Further advice on sleeping positions and on choice of beds will be found in Chapter 6.)

3. For the first two or three days lie as quietly as possible, taking meals in bed and only moving to go to the toilet.

4. Care will be needed in getting out of bed, in order to avoid unnecessary pain. A description of the best way to minimize the discomfort is given in Chapter 6.

5. Moving around in a normal upright position may be impossible, so forget your pride and crawl on all fours to and from the toilet.

6. Avoid using the bath, as one slip could aggravate or restart your pain. Either take a shower or settle for a wash-down using a hand basin or bowl.

7. Going to the toilet at this time may become a more frequent occurrence, and if so this is probably due to tension. As long as you have normal control of your bladder and bowels, there is no cause for alarm. *If you find you are losing control, get in touch with your doctor at once.* Clearing your bowels can be painful because it necessitates an increase in abdominal pressure, which can irritate the cause of your back pain by pressing tissues on to the inflamed structures. It is important to avoid constipation by eating plenty of fruit and food containing roughage. Don't slouch on the toilet but sit upright. It will help if you raise the knees slightly higher than the hips by resting the feet on a low stool, a pile of books or even an empty shoebox.

8. Sit in a firm chair with good back support. Do not sit for long periods at a time, but get up and move around every fifteen minutes or so. Try to sit as naturally erect as possible with the hollow of your back supported, and again it may help to place your feet on a low stool. Some sufferers find that they cannot sit upright because of the pain and that they have to slouch in the chair to find relief. If you come into this category then make sure you provide support for your back, in whatever position you adopt.

Getting Back to Normal

At one time patients with acute back pain were often told to go and lie down on the floor and stay there for three weeks. This is of questionable value because prolonged bed rest and total lack of activity results in loss of muscle strength which is vital to normal spinal function. In addition there could be muscle wasting, changes in the circulation and some loss of calcium in the bones. The really intense pain usually settles down by the third or fourth day, and you should then start getting up for increasing lengths of time, interspersed with bed rest.

A good spinal support can be of considerable assistance at this stage, not only for comfort but because of the confidence it provides in helping you to return to normal. These are now obtainable from the larger chemists, and under certain circumstances may be supplied by a hospital or private physiotherapist, but you can make a good temporary substitute for yourself. You will need:

1. Two 6-inch-wide crepe bandages (available from your local chemist).
2. Two corrugated cardboard sheets or a box with panels no less than 30 cm (12 ins) by 20 cm (9 ins). The better the grade of box, the more effective the support you will get.
3. Some form of adhesive padding like chiropody felt or foam, no more than 10 cm (4 ins) thick. Your chemist should have this, but if not use an old piece of blanket or cotton wool.

Mark the pieces of cardboard as shown in the diagram, making sure that the corrugations run across the pad as indicated. Attach the padding to the side of the cardboard which will be placed against your body. It may be advisable to wear a pair of cotton pants between your skin and the pads to avoid excessive perspiration. Position the front pad over the lower part of your abdomen, so that the sharper end rests just above the central bony junction of the pelvis. The larger pad should be placed over the back, with the rounded bottom section in line with the top of the hip

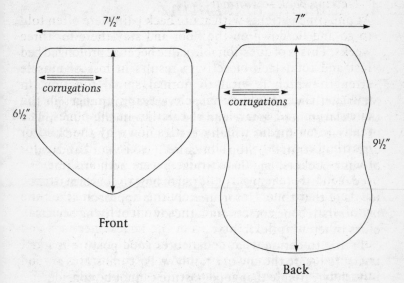

joints. Using a crepe bandage, bind the pads into position firmly but not too tightly, making sure the bandage covers the pads evenly. If they wish, women may prefer to use an old pantie girdle to keep the pads in place.

The better care you take of your back during the initial period after an acute attack the sooner you will feel better. Do not try to work your pain off, which will only make it worse – rest, support and a gradual return to activity is the safe and sensible way to a full recovery. Try to maintain a natural erect posture when sitting and standing, and avoid prolonged or sudden stooping. If you must bend, bend hips and knees and not your back. When you have got over the initial misery, begin to exercise a little each day in order to regain your fitness: seek advice from your doctor or health advisor as to which exercises are safe and beneficial. A good general rule to observe is: If it hurts, don't do it!

4 Standing and Lifting

Mention the word posture to any average group of people in the western hemisphere and they will immediately think of the rigid positions which were popular in the Victorian era. 'Sit up straight', 'Stop slouching', 'Take your hands out of your pockets' and 'Don't fidget', were admonishments used regularly to remind children of how to conform to the ideals of that time. Unfortunately this approach, like the use of whalebone corsets, took the joy out of living because of its inherent inflexibility.

Trying to define what constitutes good posture is like trying to locate the end of a rainbow. Postural states are so infinitely variable that good posture cannot be considered as some fixed stereotype. When people are being taught how to gain a better posture, they are often made to sit or stand in front of a mirror and encouraged to adopt a text-book description of a 'proper posture'. This is fine as far as it goes, but too frequently the lesson stops there, when in reality it is only the starting point from which the individual can go on to achieve a truly free-flowing dynamic use of the body. It will perhaps serve to illustrate this point, if you consider the differences between a guardsman-like stance and a child skipping through autumn leaves.

Many traditional and orthodox medicines draw heavily on the past. The ancient philosophies recognized that the mind and body were not independent but were components of a cohesive whole, a concept which is often forgotten today. Posture should be considered as the result of an interaction between mental and physical states. You might try to picture yourself, for instance, when you are walking into cold driving rain and compare it with the general bearing you would adopt on a bright warm sunny day when

all was well with your world. Think of the listless movements of a sad depressed person, or the apologetic look of
a shy and diffident one.

Good posture makes us alert and ready for action,
without being in a state of constant tension. Modern
society places substantial physiological and psychological
stresses on people which can be as taxing as any physical
burden, and this may be one of the reasons why so many
people suffer with neck and back problems related to
tension. Next time you are in a crowded train or even an
office, look around for the tell-tale hunched shoulders of
those under stress. The effects of poor posture on general
health are not fully appreciated.

Simple postural strain, when undertaking unexpected
activity – for example, having to sit for long hours on poorly
designed chairs at a conference or meeting – can lead to
general aching in the middle and lower back. Normally this
can be resolved with rest, and the only therapy that is
required is a sound night's sleep. The situation is more
complicated, however, when poor posture has become
habitual.

The symptoms in these circumstances will increase in
their intensity to the point where they can markedly
reduce the individual's level of health. In addition,
persistently poor posture creates a proneness to strains,
pains and other minor irritants, which seem to take longer
and longer to respond to treatment. In some cases, the
constant low-grade pain leads to mild depression which
may eventually escalate into an obsession with the many
and varied symptoms. Sufferers often feel guilty that there
seems to be no real proven medical cause for their
predicament. Fortunately, there is some evidence of an
increasing tendency to consider the whole person rather
than limiting attention to the physical symptoms.

Aiming for Your Own Ideal Posture

Because of the infinite variations that exist within the
human race, it is not possible to define a simple ideal for the

whole population. Basically there are three main body types. The tall thin ectomorph tends to lean forward in a top-heavy, slouched position; the mesomorph is of average height and build and should be least troubled about posture; whilst the short endomorph is likely to be over-weight and adopts a bottom-heavy posture, with an increased curve of the spine in the lumbar region. These clear-cut divisions are to an extent artificial, and most people will fall somewhere between two of them, but it is useful to be aware of the postural weaknesses of each group when considering your own postural state.

Good posture is about maintaining a correct and balanced body alignment which permits easy flowing activity for the minimum expenditure of energy and muscular effort. Human stability is based on balanced forces, and when this balance is disturbed and the component parts have lost their fine tuning, damage is more likely to occur. Although some people are fortunate and retain a well developed natural postural sense, many of us have forgotten what it feels like to be free within our bodies. In order to regain our natural birthright and be able to live in an unrestrained relaxed manner, without any tension or pain, we have to learn how to listen to what our bodies are telling us. The way to postural health is through knowledge, awareness and graded activity.

The Control of Posture

Whenever we move or adjust our position in space, we expose our bodies to the effects of the pull of gravity. These gravitational forces have to be constantly counterbalanced or we would just fall over. As well as the continual pressures, there are intermittent external forces encountered in our daily activities which can disturb our postural equilibrium.

We are fortunate that nearly all the necessary controls of posture are made at an unconscious reflex level. A very exact control is maintained by the central nervous system, which reacts to the messages it receives from the eyes, from the balance receptors in the inner ear, and from the countless tension and pressure sensors that are located in the muscles, tendons, joint capsules, ligaments and skin. Signals from various parts of the nervous system are transmitted to and activate the muscle groups that are required to equalize and therefore counteract the unbalancing forces. These controls are so precise that an absolute minimum of energy is expended to restore equilibrium. If circumstances require, the automatic controls can be overridden by conscious action.

The highly specialized patterns of reflexes which are an essential component of all movement as well as of the upright human posture are acquired during the first four years of life and built on as new skills are mastered like learning to ride a bicycle, drive a car or ski. A growing infant gradually achieves a stable upright position, first by crawling and then by standing holding on to furniture before staggering around unaided with a wide-based waddling gait. Finally, by the age of three, the child has become independent and upright. By the age of four there is sufficient confidence in its base for the child to lean over with a stooped back to pick up objects, rather than squatting down.

During this crucial period a whole network of special pathways are established within the central nervous system. The process could be likened to the programming of a computer, which permits this aspect of the body function to continue at an automatic level, leaving the conscious part of the brain free to concentrate on other important matters. If, owing to disease or injury in later life, there are disturbances to the nervous postural pathways – for example a head injury, a stroke or a broken back with damage to the spinal cord or nerve roots – it is necessary to go through a lengthy period of 're-programming' and rehabilitation before balance and possibly modified but useful gait can be regained. Unless you are unlucky enough to lose the ability to balance your body, however, it is easy to take the postural senses for granted, and to forget how important an efficient, functional posture is for general health and stability.

Standing Upright

Because the standing position is used regularly as a prelude to movement, it is important to start from the best base possible, otherwise the subsequent movement is likely to be inefficient. In order to check how your basic standing posture compares with the standard 'norm', ideally you need the help of two full-length mirrors placed at 90° to one another. A single mirror, however, will be adequate, and the elements of the standing position will be described on the assumption that only one mirror is available.

You may be surprised that when you try to adjust to your ideal natural standing posture you feel uncomfortable and even slightly deformed. This is because your mind has accepted your modified posture as the proper body image, so that as you attempt to correct your current poor position, the various soft structures of the spine that have shortened over a period of time will become stretched and send signals to this effect.

Once you have checked yourself against the standard posture, don't forget to recheck yourself when you pass any reflective surface. While you are correcting your body image, you will be exercising your conscious control to modify the faults in your unconscious postural programme. If you take things in steady stages, you should be able to achieve a reasonable posture in a very short time, without too many difficulties.

For the initial assessment, you will need to undress at least down to your underclothes, or better still to take everything off. Stand in front of the mirror and make sure you can get a clear side view of yourself from head to toe. Although it may be difficult, try as far as possible to avoid turning your head. Compare how you are standing with the standard posture and then gently try to achieve a similar one. If you find this is difficult and painful, you should not proceed until you have sought the advice of a doctor or therapist who specializes in back care.

Beginning with the feet, the weight of the body should fall just in front of the ankle joints. The angle of the ankle joint should be 90° and the knees should be straight, but not locked into a forced position. The pelvis should be lined up so that the hip joint is directly over the knee.

Now look at the rib cage, and check if it is balanced above the pelvis. It should be raised slightly so that the bottom of

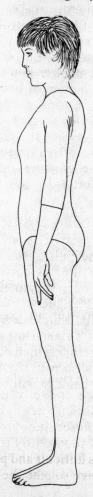

The balanced posture

the breastbone (sternum) is angled forwards and slightly outwards. Try letting your chest droop and notice the immediate reduction in the depth of breathing.

The most important section of all is the head and neck. Where the head leads the body follows, and when the head-neck relationship is incorrect, this tends to throw the rest of the spinal system into disarray. Try to bring your head back a little so that the small bony protrusions behind your ears (the mastoid processes) come into the same line as your hip joint. As you do this your chin will automatically tuck in slightly and your head will feel as if it is going upwards, taking the rest of your body with it. Notice the sensation of lightness and freedom this produces, because when the body is in a state of balance it is at its most efficient and requires minimal energy.

Once you have learned to check your posture, it will become progressively easier to maintain the new body alignment. Don't be surprised if people tell you how well you look or that you are growing younger. Do have a try. It is really worth the effort!

Working in a Standing Position

A great many daily activities are carried out from a standing position, and unless you have developed good postural habits you will be using your body in ways that may produce tension, are very inefficient, and result in cumulative stress and fatigue.

The common faults which develop include bending forwards from the waist to reach low worksurfaces, standing with the feet close together, which necessitates more trunk movements than would normally be required, and forgetting to get down to a reasonable height when working at a task around knee level.

Stooping over Low Surfaces

Typical situations often associated with poor posture are washing up, ironing, food preparation and working at a bench in the greenhouse or garage. Unless you are fortunate enough to be able to have your kitchen or workbench custom built to suit your exact dimensions, some compromise will be called for to optimize your conditions.

When washing up or preparing vegetables, try putting the bowl on top of the draining board and using the sink for the clean dishes or for the saucepan for the vegetables. Ironing can be made less tiring if the ironing board is adjusted to around waist height, and if you find this task a particular strain, a high stool may enable you to sit-stand while you are doing it.

In the garage and greenhouse the height of benches and worksurfaces is often too low. In this case try raising the supporting legs on bricks until a comfortable height is achieved, somewhere between hip and waist level. Aim to avoid standing still for more than ten minutes at a time and move around and change your activities fairly frequently.

Not many people realize that the key to efficient movement is the way in which the feet are placed. Standing with the feet too close together tends to lead to tense, restrictive trunk movements, with an increase in the amount of twisting of the spine. When standing, it is more efficient to have the feet hip-width apart as this provides a broader and more stable base. It is also useful to remember to adjust your feet to anticipate a movement, for example when moving a heavy saucepan from the cooker to an adjacent worksurface, place the feet in such a way that the weight can be transferred across from one to the other in a smooth motion.

If you have to stand for long periods at a time, the strain on your back can be relieved by placing one foot higher than the other, like the cowboy drinking at a Western bar. Changing the weight from one foot to the other every few minutes can help to spread the load.

One activity which causes those who suffer with their backs a lot of pain and irritation is leaning over a washbasin to rinse their face or hair. A logical solution is to wash your hair under a shower, but if you have no shower, some of the stress can be reduced by washing your hair over the bath

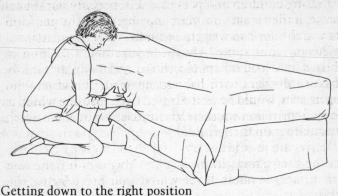

Getting down to the right position

and supporting the spine by using one arm as a strut against the bathroom wall or top edge of the bath.

To avoid stooping when making beds, cleaning the bath or dusting low shelves, and for other similar activities, get down to the proper level by either kneeling or squatting. This advice also applies to gardening. If you have problems in getting low enough, there are specially designed kneeling stools with side handles which make the task much easier. Long-handled tools and raised beds are other solutions to particular stooping problems.

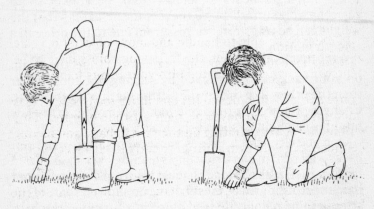

Cumulative stress . . .   . . . avoided

Handling children and pets can be especially hazardous because, if they trust you, your body becomes the platform from which they can wriggle and move, placing additional stresses on your spine. Always ensure that this kind of mobile, active load is kept close in to your body, preferably across it. Mothers with babies and young children who sleep in a cot, would be well advised to choose one which is high enough to prevent their having to stoop over too much when picking up their child.

Equally, you should not try to reach too high, particularly when holding things like washing. Always bring the line down to a reasonable level whilst you are pegging the washing out.

Handling Loads

There is every reason to believe that the human body is not designed for regular or heavy load-handling. The argument as to the safest way to move and lift objects has been going on for many years and was intensified in the early 1950s, when the concept of kinetic handling was introduced by Tom McClurg Anderson, a Scottish physiotherapist. His ideas on relating the structure of the body to safe functional activity were greeted as the solution to back pain in industry. Unfortunately, however, those teaching his techniques too often condensed his ideas into a rigid drill which did not adequately cover the varied range of circumstances in which lifting can take place.

In order to be able to handle and move objects in a safe and yet practical manner, the following points have to be appreciated and incorporated into your lifting habits.

Your approach. In order to lift and move loads safely, it is important that you have the right attitude of mind. This will include concentrating on the task in hand and having confidence in your own abilities to carry it out successfully.

Clothing. Usually the load is held close to the body. If what you are lifting is greasy, messy or distasteful, it is natural to be reluctant to hold the load close to yourself, especially when wearing good clothes. In industry protective clothing is normally provided, but choosing the proper clothes for domestic work does not always receive the attention it merits. Protective clothing should be comfortable and permit free movement. Avoid having hard, knobbly objects in trouser pockets during handling activity, as the load can easily catch on these or cause them to dig into your body. When handling rough material like timber, and metal with rough edges, make sure you wear good strong gloves, preferably with reinforced palms. Shoes for work should be sensible, with low heels, and provide support to the heel and ankle. They should also have non-slip soles. If you are a woman and have to handle loads frequently you will probably work in a more relaxed manner if you wear trousers.

Preparation. The whole area in which loads are being moved should be checked to see that it is clear of any debris which could lead to a fall. It is very easy, when working in the garden or shed, to leave tools and materials on the floor – polythene, paper and wood are commonly involved in slips, trips and falls. Also, if benches are involved, see that these too are clear.

Placing your feet properly. Whenever you handle loads it is important to have a stable base. If you keep your feet together you will be relying on a small unstable base. You should aim, therefore, to stand as close to the load as possible, your feet hip-width apart and one foot slightly in front of the other, and to keep the load between the base created by your feet.

Getting down to the load. Always try to avoid bending your spine when reaching down to get hold of a load. Your spine should be naturally erect, and not bent or twisted to one side. Your shoulders must be kept level and facing the same way as the pelvis. When it becomes necessary to reach down for a load, *bend the hips and knees until the load can be grasped with ease.* Two further points should be borne in

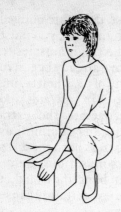

Load kept between base
of feet wherever possible

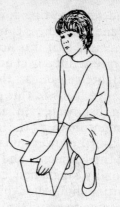

Test the load and tip
it to get a better lift

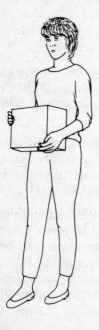

Hold the load close
to the body

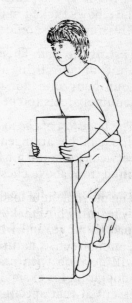

Ideal lifting position
for heavier loads, between
knee and hip height

mind when getting down to a load. First, if you are obliged to bend your knees completely to reach the load, you must appreciate that it is not possible for the thigh muscles to operate at full power until the knees have already begun to straighten by at least three inches. Many of us, when trying to move loads in this position, tend to lean forwards and then backwards in an attempt to generate the extra momentum to get the load moving. This can be harmful, as rocking the lower spinal vertebrae can stress both the discs and the ligaments and often leads to more serious injury. Secondly, single-handed lifting, as when handling a bucket or drum, should be avoided as it will almost certainly cause the spine to be rotated or bent sideways.

Holding the load. Never rely on fingertips when holding a load but always try to grasp the object with the whole hand, particularly the palms and root of the fingers. Try to keep the elbows tucked in to the side of your body and so avoid stressing your shoulders and neck muscles.

Testing the load. There is only one person who knows the limits of your lifting abilities – yourself. Learn to listen to your body and don't proceed to lift anything which genuinely feels too heavy or too bulky.

The position of the load. Loads are best handled, wherever this can be arranged, when they are initially located between knee and hip height. They are most difficult when lifted from above chest height and from floor level.

The movement of loads can be made much safer and easier by learning how make best use of your body, how to get the load to move, and what lifting aids can assist you best. Common sense, natural balance, co-ordination and timing will develop with practice – although they will not be enough in, for example, industry and nursing, where it is essential that specific techniques should be learned and absorbed.

5 *Sitting Pretty*

The lifting and handling of heavy loads is often assumed to be the main cause of back injuries, but there is growing evidence that the way we sit may be another significant factor. Comparative studies of people who live uncomplicated lives in so-called primitive societies and of those who live in the developed countries have shown that back problems are much less common among the 'natural' group, and it may well be that differences in sitting posture could be contributory to this. Since members of undeveloped societies use little or no furniture, most people are obliged to squat or sit cross-legged, and in this position the lumbar spine is either flattened or curved slightly outwards. Most of the body weight is taken by the bones of the leg, thigh and pelvis and very little stress is placed on the ligaments of the spine. Those who adopt this position seem to be able to stay in it for long periods.

Sitting in chairs is essentially an unnatural habit which many of us are forced to adopt from a very early age. As it is highly unlikely that we will revert to squatting or sitting cross-legged on the floor, it is essential that we understand about the best ways in which to sit, and then ensure that what we sit on, and at, is designed to meet our postural needs.

Learning to Sit in Comfort

The fixed ideas of the Victorian period, and even earlier, about the way a well bred person should behave meant that sitting up straight was, and generally still is, considered to be the ideal. Unfortunately this upright position is far from natural, and when adopted for long periods can lead to fatigue and cumulative stress. Unless the chairs we use for either work or leisure are properly designed to provide the right degree of freedom of movement and adequate support, we can soon end up with backache.

The ideal seated posture is one in which you are able to relax or work without any perceptions of pain, stress, strain or fatigue. The various body segments should be supported in such a way that muscular activity is kept to a minimum and the ligaments and muscles are not placed under unnecessary tension. As with standing, however, the ideal is not easy to define, both because of the variety of reasons why we sit – for work, relaxation, driving, pleasure, etc. – and because of the many conflicting theories that are currently being proposed. Again, look around you and see how people sit on the bus or train, when watching television, writing a letter or working at a machine in a factory. The way we sit is influenced to a great extent by the furniture we are using, but also by how we are feeling at a particular time.

My own experience of working with back pain sufferers and observing school children suggests that there should be no hard-and-fast rules about this or that type of posture. Provided furniture which corresponds to the individual's needs is available, everyone should be able to select the most comfortable position for themselves, once they have been given enough information and guidance to form the basis of a reasoned judgment. Obviously, really dreadful slouching or ramrod rigid positions should be actively discouraged.

Other relevant factors which also require attention are efficient lighting, in which the match of natural and artificial light is carefully balanced to avoid glare, and the basic consideration of correcting poor eyesight.

Some General Concepts

Before you can begin your search for a sound and comfortable seated position, you will need to know not only what you are trying to achieve, but the mechanics of sitting and some of the latest thinking on the subject.

When you sit, the weight of the upper trunk, arms and

pelvis is supported on the two bony protrusions in your buttocks known as the ischeal tuberosities. If you feel them, you will discover that each one is about the size of the first segment of your thumb. As is probably obvious, trying to balance the body on these two lumps alone is very difficult, and additional support has to be provided by the thighs and back. There are three basic positions for sitting, from which all other positions are derived – although none of these is without its disadvantages.

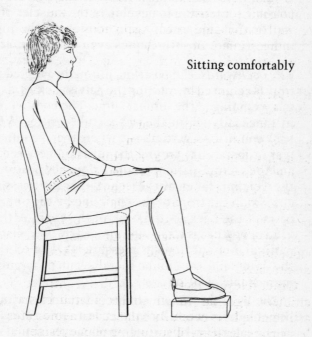

Sitting comfortably

The standard position is one in which the weight of the trunk is directly over the buttocks and thighs, and the lumbar curve can become flattened as the position is affected by gravity. This position can create tension in the back muscles and ligaments in the lumbar area and mechanically there could be increased loading on the spine.

The forward lean position, usually considered to be associated with activity or attention, is adopted when writing at a desk or working at a flat surface. The pelvis is tipped forward by bending the hip, and the body weight falls in front of the ischeal tuberosities and may cause the lumbar spine to arch forwards. Because the position is basically unstable, the upper spinal muscles are brought into action to help stabilize the head and this leads to fatigue and tension in the region of the neck and upper arms. If pressure is taken on the free arm when writing or drawing, it is possible for tension to develop in the muscles of the chest wall on that side, causing a pain which may be mistaken for indigestion or in severe cases even for a heart attack.

The backwards lean position, normally adopted for relaxation, is achieved by rotating the pelvis backwards, resulting in a rounding of the lumbar spine. The body weight in this instance falls behind the ischeal tuberosities. With certain back conditions, particularly where there is some wear and tear or instability around the junction between the spine and the sacrum, patients adopt a slouched posture in which the weight is taken by the ischeal tuberosities, sacrum and coccyx on the front of the chair and by the upper and mid parts of the back on the back of the chair. Although this kind of posture is often discouraged by therapists, in these particular circumstances pressure is taken off the joint of the spine and the lumbo-sacral segment is pulled into a more stable position.

There are three main groups of structures which have to be considered when looking at seated postures. These are the intervertebral discs and vertebrae, the spinal ligaments, and the muscles of the back and thighs.

The discs in the lower lumbar region are loaded even in a normal relaxed sitting position and, as a result of increased leverage effects, these pressures build up as the spine becomes more and more curved when the trunk has to lean forwards, for example in working at a desk. In this position the vertebrae are forced together at the front and separated at the back, which then tends to place the spinal ligaments and associated soft structures under tension. Because the body has to adopt a position away from its normal vertical line, the spinal muscles are obliged to work in order to prevent it from falling forward. This effort can easily result in fatigue and general aching in the whole area of the spine.

Different studies into the pressure within the discs, positions of least muscular effort and general posture all seem to indicate that when the angle between the trunk and the thigh at the front of the body is between 105° and 120°, then the muscles around the hip joint are relaxed, the pressure on the intervertebral discs is lowered and the natural curve of the lumbar spine is maintained.

Sitting Down

Most of us never give a second thought to how we sit down. We walk into a room and just dump ourselves in a seat and then expect our bodies to adapt to it. The results of this in the long term can be posturally harmful. When sitting down you should try to guide your hips and buttocks right into the junction of the chair back and seat, and then sit down by moving the hips downards and forwards into the final position. This method tends to prevent slouching and sliding forwards, as this will be resisted by the friction between the clothing and skin, and the fabric of the chair. The more normal method of sitting, where the hips are pushed backwards as they contact the chair, acts in the reverse way and is far less efficient, as the buttocks and back do not come into full contact with the back of the chair, and the body is allowed to slide forward.

Sitting at Work

By now it will be obvious that trying to achieve a seated work posture which takes account of all the relevant considerations is not easy (and is almost impossible when driving, though back and head supports can help).

As we gain a better understanding of the spine, many of the previously held beliefs about the ideal work posture are being questioned. The new ideas that are emerging promise to be very exciting and beneficial to those who are obliged to sit for long periods as part of their daily routine. Two solutions have been suggested for achieving the 'ideal' position, one involving a seat which slopes forwards and the other a chair with a backrest which tilts backwards to the particular angle required by the individual.

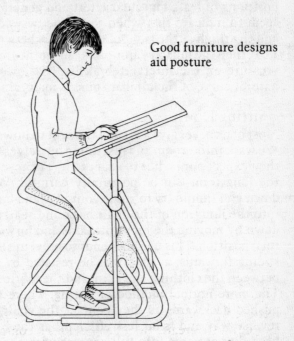

Good furniture designs aid posture

The forward-tilting chair was a concept developed in Scandinavia as early as the late 1960s. One of the leaders in this movement was Dr A. C. Mandal. As a result of observing children in school, who often tipped their chairs forward on to the front legs in order to improve their working position, he developed the concept of a chair with a forward-tilting seat and desks with sloping tops which were slightly higher than standard furniture. He recommended that the seat should be able to tilt forward to an angle of 20° away from the horizontal, and that the front edge of the chair should be between 5 cms and 10 cms above the height of the kneecap – i.e. 49 – 60 cms from the ground for the average adult. The desk that goes with this chair should be somewhere between 80 cms and 90 cms high depending on the dimensions of the user. (Note that a standard office desk is around 74 cms high and has a flat top.) It is now possible to obtain a number of commercial products which conform to these recommendations.

An alternative solution to the problem, specifically designed for people working with visual display units (VDUs), was suggested by Ettienne Grandjean, an ergonomist at the Swiss Federal Institute of Technology. Grandjean and his colleagues developed an adjustable work-station which was tried by sixty-eight VDU operators. The position of the screen and keyboard height were adjusted by means of an electric motor, and the distance and angle of the screen was manually controlled by the operator. The chair that went with the work-station was fully adjustable, including the angle of the backrest to the seat. When the preferred working positions of the people in the trial were checked, it was found that many of the previous recommendations made for VDU stations differed from those chosen by the operators. Those in the research programme selected higher keyboard heights, reduced viewing angles and sat with their chair backrests adjusted between 91° and 120° with an average setting of 104°. This is around 10° greater than the previous recommended back-to-seat angle.

Car Seats

Because of the need for car manufacturers to fit the dimensions of a wide range of sizes and shapes and yet permit all-round visibility, it is probably quite surprising that in general car seats do manage to be reasonably comfortable. Inevitably, though, the degree of comfort is very variable. In one large company where there were a number of lorries of different makes in the delivery fleet,

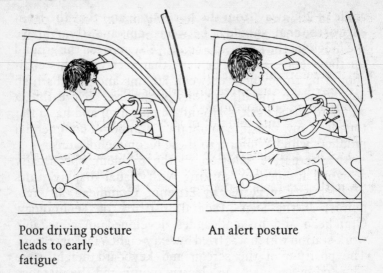

Poor driving posture
leads to early
fatigue

An alert posture

the drivers had to be issued with personal back supports in
one type of lorry because the seats were so badly designed.
A sales representative in the same company suddenly
developed back pain for no apparent reason. When his past
history was checked, it was discovered that the only thing
that was different in his life was that he had changed his car
a week earlier. The simple expedient of a new seat
completely resolved his back pain.

If you are a back pain sufferer and find that your car seat
is not as comfortable as you would wish, you may well be
able to ease the problem by buying one of the specially
designed supports which are available.

Home Comforts

When choosing furniture for the home, there are bound to
be other criteria as well as simple comfort. Personal tastes,
decor, lifestyle, not to mention price, have to be taken into
consideration, and while the ideal chair would be adjustable
to suit the needs of each individual user, this is hardly very
realistic. However, a number of manufacturers do produce
chairs which embody many of the ideal design elements.

When looking at furniture for relaxation, do not only consider the look but also, and more importantly, test it out properly. Ask yourself some relevant questions:

- Is it comfortable to sit in?
- Is your back supported properly or does the seat force you into a poor position?
- Can you get into and out of the seat easily, or is it too narrow or too wide?
- Does the upholstery give sufficiently to accommodate your body or is it too hard or too soft?
- Are the arm rests in the right place to enable you to sit down and get up in a good relaxed position, whatever you are doing?
- Are you sure you are buying a chair which is genuinely suited to your needs, that not only looks good but is good for *you*, the user?

The use of chairs is an unnatural habit adopted by our civilization, and the time spent in a sitting position seems to be on the increase. Poor seated posture must be considered to be a major contributory factor to modern back pain problems, and it is important therefore first to try to reduce the time spent seated and then, if you have to sit, to select a well designed chair and make sure you adopt a good position.

Perhaps more than anything else, it is important that our children are permitted to use their bodies properly during their formative years, and are not forced into unhealthy postural habits by their school, or other, furniture. There is enough information available to designers and manufacturers to enable them to develop furniture that is beneficial to the users, but it is up to you, the customer, to encourage the manufacture of the best and most suitable products.

6 *Sleep and Relaxation*

The importance of proper sleep for personal well-being cannot be over stressed. It is vital both for restoring energy and drive and for repairing the tissues of the body, and lack of it is likely to be among the more distressing and frustrating consequences of back injury. The quality of sleep depends upon general health, a relaxed mind, regular habits and a good bed, though the actual amount each person requires will vary – it is claimed that some world leaders have been able to survive on three or four hours a night, aided by catnaps during the day.

Normal sleep contains two separate phases, orthodox sleep and dreaming sleep, with five periods of orthodox sleep, of equal length, interspersed with five periods of dreaming sleep which become progressively longer. During dreaming sleep the body relaxes totally, and if your bed is too soft or too hard the various joints of the body can become strained and distorted.

In the course of an average night, it is also normal to change position up to fifty times. If you share a bed with another person, the problems this can create are fairly obvious unless the bed is wide enough to allow two people reasonable space in which to move.

In order to re-establish normal sleeping patterns, if these have been in any way disturbed, it will be helpful to know a little more about sleeping positions and about the very important subject of beds.

Sleeping Positions

There are two sleeping postures used by humans living in a natural state. The first is lying on the side in a curled position with an arm under the head as a pillow. An alternative is lying flat on the back with the head supported by some kind of headrest. Were we to lie in any one position for any length of time, we would soon end up with areas of soreness over the hips, sacrum or other body points. Those who suffer from back pain may turn into a position which causes their pain to increase, and this will result in further loss of sleep. Three basic positions can help to ease back pain and encourage relaxation and sleep.

On the Back. Place two pillows under the head and a bolster or two pillows, firmly rolled in a towel, under the thighs. This arrangement helps to keep the hips in a bent position and relaxes the small tight psoas muscles which run from the lumbar spine over the front of the thighs.

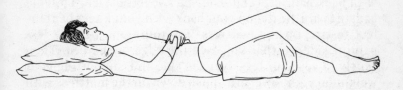

Lying on the Side. Lie on the side which causes less pain, with enough pillows under the head to provide support for the neck. Because the upper leg is inclined to fall across and down over the lower one, this can place a twisting strain on the pelvis and lower back. The strain can be eliminated by placing a pillow between the knees or using one of the specially designed foam pads like the 'knee bean' which is not quite as bulky as a pillow.

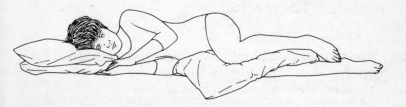

Extended Side-Lying. For those who prefer to lie more on their front, place a pillow under the chest and trunk and hug it as a child hugs a teddy bear. This serves to prevent you rolling right over on to your face.

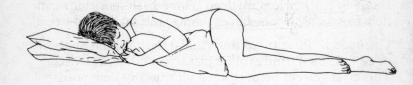

Getting out of Bed

Getting out of bed can sometimes be difficult for those with back pain, especially during a severe attack. To avoid causing pain, lie flat on your back with your knees bent up, feet resting on the mattress. Try rolling on to your less painful side, so that you face the edge of the bed. Then gently lower your legs over the side and, supporting your weight on your lower arm, push down on the mattress with your other arm to get you into a sitting position.

Once you are upright, support your trunk by placing your hands on the mattress about 6 – 8 inches away from you, and use your arms to brace the spine. To stand up, lean slightly forward, pushing on your hands as you begin to straighten your knees and hips. In both sitting and standing, try to keep the spine fixed, as if it were a stiff rod. The procedure may be reversed to get back into bed.

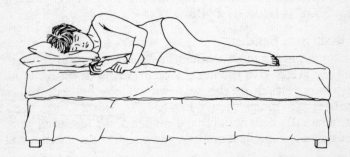

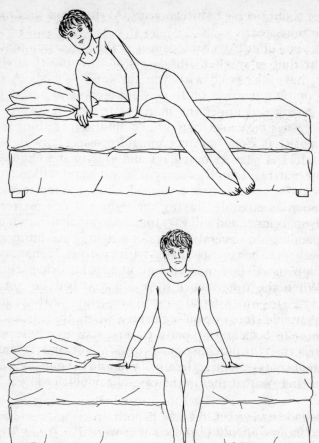

Beds and Bedding

Although many of us spend at least a third of our lives in bed, we rarely give the necessary attention to this item of furniture, either in the way we select our beds or in bothering to renew them when they are worn. Contrary to the generally held belief that a good bed will last a lifetime, beds, even of the best quality, show signs of wear and tear after about twelve to fifteen years. At this stage they need to be changed.

If you suffer from back pain it is almost certain that at some time or another your doctor or other health adviser will have discussed with you the topic of beds. A not uncommon instruction to new sufferers is to put an old door or board under the mattress to firm it up. As an emergency measure this is often helpful, but as a long-term proposition it is not recommended, especially if your mattress is past its best days and sags in the middle. If your mattress is in this sorry state no board will make it any better and it is time to consider buying a replacement as soon as possible. Buying the right bed is a matter of personal choice and will vary from individual to individual, depending on several factors – weight, size, build and whether the bed is to be shared with a partner. Proneness to back pain will be a most important added consideration.

When the time comes to buy a new bed, do not be tempted to go for a bargain just to save money. Always go to a reputable store or bedding centre, where there is a wide choice of beds and properly trained staff to advise you. Never rush the purchase of a bed, take your time, try out a number of types and styles until you find the one that suits you (and your partner in the case of a double bed.)

What to Look for in a Bed

A good bed should provide your body with a reasonable degree of support, permit you to lie in a natural position and promote relaxation and sleep. The mattress and base should be firm enough to prevent your body sinking, but not so hard that it will not accommodate your hip and shoulder and gently support the hollow of your waist.

You will have noticed the words 'firm' and 'hard' being used to describe mattresses; a firm bed suits most users but a hard bed will prove uncomfortable for all but a limited number. Some manufacturers use the term 'orthopaedic type' as an indication that they are specially designed for those with back problems. Though there are several

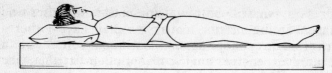

Too hard

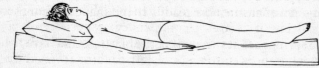

Too soft

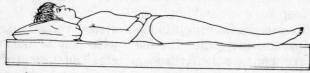

Just right

excellent 'orthopaedic type' beds on the market, the use of the term 'orthopaedic' in itself provides no guarantee that the bed in question has any special medical qualities or that it will cure your back problems. This does not mean that a good bed will not help to reduce the problem of back pain – there are people whose problems have been completely resolved once they changed their worn-out old bed for a new one.

The size of the bed is another important consideration. Always make sure that the bed you buy is nine inches longer than the tallest user, and a double bed should be at least five feet wide if both occupants are to have sufficient room to sleep and move naturally.

Mattresses

A bed consists of two key components, the mattress and base. Mattresses can vary considerably in type and construction, from spring interior to foam; even horsehair mattresses can still be found in some farmhouses and cottages. Spring-interior mattresses may have either a series of single open springs or a continuous coiled wire. In the more expensive single-coil spring mattresses, the springs are located in pockets of calico or a synthetic fabric. Each type of mattress has its own characteristics and the pocket-spring type is almost certainly the best buy, as the springs can conform more readily to the shape and contours of the sleeper.

The springs are at the heart of the mattress and have to be sandwiched between layers of felt padding, topped by a softer layer of wool or synthetic fluffed fibres which are enclosed in a ticking of padded patterns during the final sewing process. A modern alternative is to use layers of foam instead of felt and fibre.

Mattresses made entirely of foam all have the advantage of being non-allergenic. The foam used may be natural latex or chemical polyurethane mixtures, and the mattress is constructed from layers of foam of different thicknesses and densities. Recent research has indicated that the top layer should have a 10–30 per cent compression factor.

Water beds, whilst they can be very comfortable, are not only expensive but tend to provide passive rather than active support. The main disadvantage of a water bed is the sheer weight of water which the bed contains. Before considering buying one of these beds it is important to check that your floors can support the weight and that you can move the bed, should the need arise.

Bed Bases

When you think of changing your mattress have a good look at the base to make sure it is in good condition. If you place an expensive mattress on to a worn base it will be false economy, resulting in uneven wear and a ruined mattress in a matter of months.

There are many satisfactory alternatives available, from the fully sprung edge versions which provide even support over the whole base area, to the solid bases and the slatted versions as found on the pine and beech-framed beds which are popular in Northern Europe and Scandinavia. The height of the base is generally pre-set by the manufacturer but if you have a choice, a base which is roughly in line with your knee joint should make getting out of bed easier.

When buying a new bed exercise the same level of care that you would when buying a new car. Test and try a number of beds before making up your mind and if in doubt ask for expert advice. Always bear in mind that your bed will have to last up to 45,000 sleeping hours. Finally, if your partner finds your preferred choice of mattress uncomfortable, it is now possible to purchase twin beds, of different degrees of firmness. These can be zipped together to make a double bed.

Relaxation

The value of relaxation and its use to reduce stress and tension has been recognized by succeeding civilizations. In a number of religions, great emphasis is placed on the attainment of a state of inner calm by various techniques of meditation and contemplation. One of the more popular methods used in the West, which has been borrowed from the East, is Hatha yoga. Those who practise yoga will recognize many of the exercises and relaxation techniques described in this book.

The growing realization that stress, particularly when associated with the pace of our modern lifestyle, is a contributory factor in a variety of complaints, including strokes, heart disease and nervous breakdowns, has led to an increase of interest in relaxation techniques as an antidote which is both natural and inexpensive. For the back sufferer, who is plagued by muscle tension and pain, relaxation – though it will not produce a cure – can provide welcome relief and significantly aid the process of recovery.

Relaxation and activity are simply the opposite ends of the same functional pattern. Unfortunately, many people today have lost the natural ability to relax and have to be taught how to do so and allow themselves to withdraw from the killing pace of life for a few vital minutes. Relaxation is not just a matter of 'letting go' and becoming floppy, it requires conscious effort, involving both mind and body. Some people find it difficult to relearn this natural art, but once you are able to relax at will, it is possible to shut off and top up your depleted reserves in virtually any situation except the few (like driving a car) that demand your total concentration. The benefits that relaxation bring are numerous and include:

- The ability to be in total control of oneself.
- Improved health and vigour.
- Greater energy reserves and the ability to use your energy in the most economical way.
- A general reduction in heart rate and lowered blood pressure.
- A return to a more natural state which does not require the assistance of artificial stimulants or relaxants.
- Greater confidence and a quieter response to stressful situations.
- Peace of mind which leads to clarity of thought and more self-awareness and assurance.

Learning to Relax

Please read right through this section before trying it out. There are various methods which will enable you to relax your body and eventually lead to peace of mind. However, although some people in the West have mastered the mystic Eastern systems, which are based on looking into oneself or losing oneself in the vastness of the Universe, most lesser mortals have to rely on learning to relax the various muscle groups in the body in a sequence which starts at the toes and ends with the eyes. Whatever technique you try, you should not be disheartened if you do not get instant results. It may take some weeks to become really proficient.

Before attempting to relax, it is necessary to set the scene, because you can never hope to achieve a relaxed state in the middle of the bustle and noise of daily routines.

(Later, perhaps much later, you will be able to 'opt out' in spite of minor distractions.) During your period of learning to relax, find a warm, airy room, in which the light can be softened to a pleasing glow. The first few sessions will probably be the most difficult and your progress will depend on how rapidly you acquire the ability to unwind. There can be no set time or pattern to the way you learn to relax, and progress will vary from one person to another, so have patience.

First stage. Once you have selected your room you will need a rug to lie on, a pillow or folded towel on which to rest your head and possibly two more towels to place under your knees and in the hollow of your back. Lie on your back on the rug which has been placed on the floor, before pulling the pillow or folded towel under your head and neck, so that it is supported in a neutral position. Your chin should not poke forwards nor should your head tilt backwards. If you wish, place a folded towel or a pillow under your knees to provide support and to aid relaxation of the muscles over the front of your hip joints. Should you find you have a small hollow at the bottom of your spine, roll up the other towel and use it to give gentle support to this area. Move each support around until you are really comfortable. Place your arms slightly away from your body with the elbows half bent, resting your hands on the floor in the position that feels easy.

For the first two or three minutes do not do anything but mentally explore your body to see if there are any particular areas of tension or pain. These are likely to be in muscles of your neck or lower back and even in the hands and fingers, which may be clenched. At this stage, if you are not absolutely sure what 'relaxed' means, try the following routine:

1. Clench your hands to make a fist and close them tighter and tighter as you count up to 10. When you reach 10, you may be surprised at the amount of tension that has developed in your whole body.

2. Let your hands open slowly, like a flower gently uncurling, and linger over the feeling of ease that results. Try a long yawn as well.
3. Go through the tension routine twice more and then just lie quietly, letting your mind drift as it pleases.

This exercise should be sufficient for your first exploration of relaxation.

Second Stage. If at all possible, make time for your second period of relaxation on the next day, when you can take yourself into the actual relaxation techniques. Having settled down, go through the tension-relaxation routine for three or four minutes and then lie still. This time start to concentrate on your breathing. As you breathe in, picture a balloon being blown up. Fill your lungs right down to the very bottom, expanding your ribs at the same time for a count of 4. At this point sigh your breath out for a count of 6 or 7 and keep thinking of the balloon as it deflates and crumples up. Repeat this procedure 5 times and you should find that as you breathe in, the tension is more noticeable but becomes much less as you breathe out. You have now reached the stage where you can start to build on the experience of relaxation and of the effects of deep breathing on tension which you have gained so far.

Third Stage. From this point on, once you have settled yourself comfortably, go into your breathing routine, drawing the air in to fill your lungs and then sighing it out. Do not try to feel or deliberately look for the tension, but if it is present recognize it for what it is, something that can be eased away. On each outbreath, let your whole body relax a little more, until you feel yourself sinking deeper and deeper into the surface you are lying on. Let your imagination have its freedom and think of warm pink clouds which wrap around and enfold you. Keep this up for ten to twenty minutes and if you fall asleep don't worry. This is perfectly natural.

As you become more proficient, let your breathing go into an automatic state and once you have achieved total

relaxation, let your mind drift at will, as long as the ir
are pleasant and refreshing. If you find yourself begi
to think about day-to-day worries, then revert to con;
deep-breathing routines until a more peaceful stat
been regained. At the end of each session do not jun
straight away, but count backwards from 10 to one, sl
as you prepare your mind and body for normal action.
your time and try to retain the benefits of your peri
relaxation for as long as possible.

On a practical note, because you won't be able to
how to relax and practise the techniques at the same ti
it is a good idea if possible either to ask a friend to read
chapter to you or better still to tape it for yourself, reading
the text at a steady rate. Alternatively there are relaxation
tapes available for purchase, and in some areas relaxation
classes are organized by the local Back Pain Association
groups.

Once mastered, relaxation can be switched on at will and
used as often as necessary. Of course, the ability to relax
does not in itself guarantee that life will suddenly cease to
have problems, but you will find yourself in a far better
position to cope with them, and in a more controlled
manner. For back pain sufferers, relaxation offers a natural
method of pain and tension control and helps eliminate the
need for drugs and other forms of analgesia. Especially
taking into account the general health benefits it confers, it
is an art that is well worth the small effort required to
master it.

Alexander Technique – The Relaxed Revolutionary Postural System

The last few years have seen an increase in the popularity
of the Alexander Technique, and in the number of teachers
of this system of relaxed living. The technique is not
simply a therapeutic system, but embodies a whole new
lifestyle. Its postural and philosophical principles have
enabled many back pain sufferers not only to become free

of pain but to learn to control their body posture and function in every situation.

F. Matthias Alexander, the creator of this unique approach to self-awareness, was born in Tasmania in 1869 and eventually began to earn his living by reciting Shakespeare on the stage. Initially he enjoyed success, but later his career was threatened by chronic nose and throat irritation, which responded only to rest. He was assured that there was no organic explanation for his condition, and so he set about examining himself in minute detail, observing his body actions while reciting.

He soon noticed that as he started to recite he pulled his head back, at the same time drawing his breath in through his mouth and depressing his larynx, creating a gasping sound. Further examination of himself revealed that this was not a local problem but a reflection of his whole body image and poor postural habits.

Alexander assumed that these were easily corrected and that all that was necessary was to return to natural patterns of activity, but he found that this was not the case. He discovered that, far from being beneficial, many of the so-called natural postural habits contained tension components that were harmful, particularly in their effect on the relationship between the head and neck. In order to develop his technique, Alexander was obliged to discard the existing ideas of 'good posture', which tended to be based on a static or even statuesque pose, and it was only over a number of years that he was gradually able to evolve his approach to better body use and a more healthy relaxed lifestyle.

The Alexander Technique views the body and mind as a total psycho-physical organism and considers that the conscious mind can change the subconscious patterns of muscular usage. The key to the new body awareness advocated by Alexander is proper head and neck alignment as an initiator of total balanced posture, and most people who become involved in this approach visit one of the growing number of approved teachers who are to be found in most parts of the country. (Several books are also available for those who would first like to find out more about the subject for themselves.)

After an initial discussion and explanation of the concepts of the technique, there will follow a period of assessment and observation, which will continue throughout all treatment sessions. Your teacher will help you to experience a balanced relaxed posture and to relate this to achieving 'normal function' in your daily activities. As the old harmful and stress-filled habits are replaced by the new balanced postural control techniques, it is likely that you will gain an enhanced postural sense and feeling of control over yourself, a greater freedom from strain, as well as increased vigour.

Relaxation is, of course, only part of the spectrum of living. Equal emphasis must be placed on activity and exercise, and to these we shall now turn.

7 Exercise and Back Pain

The maintenance of a reasonable state of fitness, in the context of back pain, is every bit as important as the ability to relax. Not only will it reduce the likelihood of injury in the first place, but if you are unfortunate enough to suffer damage to your back it will greatly increase the chances of a rapid return to normal.

Although rest is among the most frequently prescribed treatments, and there is nothing wrong in resting until the initial severe pain has settled down, too much rest will result in loss of muscle tone and possibly a loss of mobility and overall confidence.

Exercise is a little like medicine, in that it should be tailored to the individual's needs, and the amount carefully controlled. Too much can be harmful and too little a waste of time. The practice of handing out standard lists of exercises without personal instruction is at best unwise and at worst could do harm or cause unnecessary pain so that the whole programme may be abandoned in disgust. The routine that follows is designed to enable you to progress within the limits set by your condition. It requires you to monitor what your body is telling you, and to respond in an appropriate manner.

Before you start any programme of exercises, it is generally safer to check with your doctor or therapist, particularly if you have more than just moderate pain or have any doubts. The aim of any exercise routine for back pain should be to:

- Improve the strength and tone of the key groups of muscles in the back, abdomen, thighs and buttocks.
- Gradually build up the general standard of fitness.

- Increase the range of pain-free movement and restore normal functions.
- Remove the fear of pain and boost self-confidence.

Certain basic guidelines have to be followed if you want to gain the maximum benefit from your efforts:

- Do your exercises regularly and try to set aside a small part of each day to give yourself time to go through them, and to allow yourself to relax at the end of the session.
- Do not continue with any exercise which produces an increase in your pain. Many people work under the misguided belief that treatment must hurt before it does any good.
- When you start to exercise do only 3 or 4 different exercises until you feel able to progress on to a few more. The following programme has been planned with this in mind.
- In order to prevent yourself becoming overtired and therefore possibly damaging already weakened structures, don't try to do too many of each exercise. Three of any particular exercise will usually be sufficient. As a general rule, your exercises should leave you refreshed, not washed out.
- Perform each exercise in a smooth, rhythmical manner so that you can maintain total control, breathing easily all the time. It is better not to do an exercise at all than to rush through it.
- As you feel yourself getting fitter, move on to the more advanced routines, but do only 10 exercises at any one time. If you can, try to do your exercises twice a day. Later on it should be possible for you to reduce your formal exercises to a minimum maintenance routine, going on to other forms of activity which give you pleasure, such as walking, swimming, cycling and dancing.
- Remember always to start and finish your exercise session with a simple warm-up and cool-down routine, ending with a final period of relaxation.

Exercise Routine

The equipment you will need is basically the same as that required for relaxation, i.e. a blanket or mat to lie on, a pillow or folded towel for your head, and pillows and a folded towel for your final relaxation period.

Begin with the first set of exercises and DO NOT proceed to the second and subsequent sets until you have been able to manage the first set without any stress, discomfort or marked fatigue.

Set I – Limbering Up

1. Lie down on your back on the folded blanket or mat you have placed on the floor. Place a pillow under your head and put your arms down by the sides of your body, bending your knees mid-way, so that your feet can rest comfortably on the floor. Before beginning any exercise just let your mind go into freewheel and relax the tension out of your whole system using the deep breathing routine you learned for relaxation.

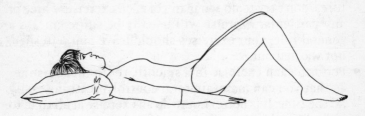

2. The next stage in the opening and closing routine is to loosen up 'key' parts of the body. As you lie on the mat try to will your head to grow away from your feet. Then turn your face fully towards your left shoulder, then towards your right shoulder, before returning to a comfortable mid-position. Repeat twice more. Now shrug your shoulders right up to your ears, then let them down, reaching with your hands as far down towards your knees as possible before coming back to the position of rest. Do this twice more.

Keeping in the same position slide the heel of your right foot towards your buttock, as far as it will go without pain, and then push the foot back down until your knee is straight. Repeat the exercise with the left foot and repeat twice more with each foot to complete 3 full exercises.

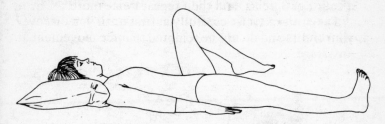

The routine so far should be done on each occasion you exercise, starting with relaxation and limbering up and then finishing after any other exercises with limbering up and relaxation in reverse order.

3. Keeping to the basic start position described in the first exercise do this next exercise without holding your breath. Imagine you have a large orange between your knees, which you are going to squeeze by tightening up your inner thigh muscles. As you squeeze, draw in your pelvic floor, abdominal and buttock muscles, which should cause your pelvis to tilt forwards and flatten your back against the floor. Hold for a count of 1 and 2 and 3 then slowly relax. Do the exercise 3 times in all.

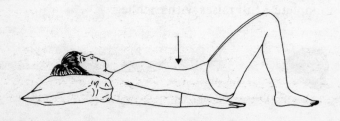

4. Turn on to your less painful side. Keep your knees and ankles together and draw your knees up towards your chest, curling up into a 'C' shape, pulling the knees and head together. Hold for a count of 3 and then slowly uncurl, stretching your legs as far as they will go, pointing the toes and slightly bowing the back. Hold for a count of 3, relax, and then repeat twice more.

Take this exercise carefully at first until you discover your limits and do not be tempted to force movement at any stage.

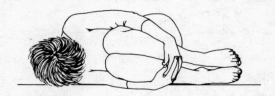

As this is the end of the first set of exercises, go back to exercises 2 and 1, and then relax for 5 minutes.

Set II – Getting a Little Stronger
This set of exercises is designed to strengthen your trunk and leg muscles. First, go through the exercises in Set I up to No. 4 and then add as many of exercises 5 – 7 as you can manage before going into the 'wind-down' routine.

5. Lie on your front if you are able, resting your head on your folded arms. Gently press your left hip into the surface you are lying on, and keeping your knee straight, raise your foot 3 inches from the floor. Hold and then lower before repeating the exercise with the right leg. Complete 3 full raises with each leg.

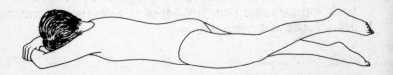

6. Remaining in the same position, breathing deeply and steadily, brace your buttock muscles and tense the trunk muscles as if trying to pull your pelvis and ribs together. Hold for a count of 3. Relax and then repeat twice more.
7. Lie on your left side and bend your left leg sufficiently to give you some support. Keeping your right leg straight, raise it away from the midline of your body as far as it will go with comfort, then return to the starting position. Repeat this 4 more times before turning over to do the same exercise on the other side.

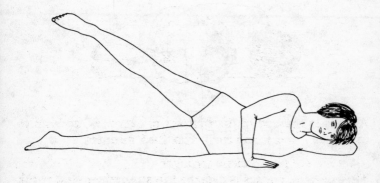

Set III – Moving On
Exercises 8 to 10 should help you to increase the range of pain-free movement in your hips and spine. Take your time and don't be tempted to use speed to get you through a movement; a smooth and steady action is the secret. Set III should be added to Sets I and II.

8. Kneel on all fours, keeping the arms and legs at 90° to your body. Gently hollow your back and raise your head to look upwards, and then go into a position with your back rounded and your head tucked in between your arms. Pause and repeat twice.

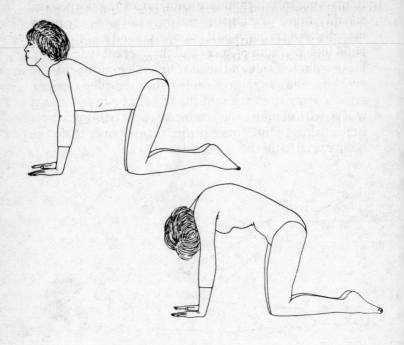

9. From the basic all fours position, bring your right knee forward to touch your left wrist. Put the leg back to the start position and repeat with the left leg. Finish 3 full exercises.

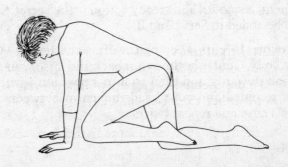

10. Adopt the position below. Keeping the hands still, push an imaginary pea with your nose as far forwards as possible. Then gently return to the start position to push the next pea. Push 3 peas altogether.

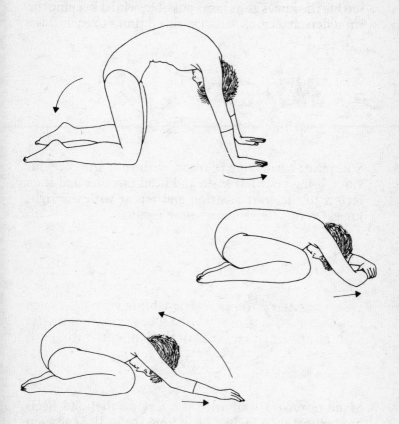

Additional Exercises

You have now reached the end of Set III, and should you wish to add more exercises – either mobilizing exercises to substitute for other exercises in Set II, or strengthening exercises for others in Set III – you may do so. Always remember, though, never to do more than 10 exercises in any daily routine.

Mobilizing Exercises

1. Lie on your back with your knees bent and the soles of the feet resting on the floor. Keeping the knees together, swing your legs first to the right and then to the left, letting the knees go as far as possible, whilst keeping the shoulders and trunk still. Do this 3 times to each side.

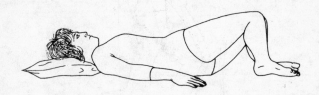

2. Still in the basic lying position, with your arms by your sides, bring your left knee and head together and then return to the start position and repeat with the right knee. Do this twice more before resting.

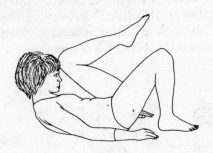

3. Stand against a wall with the feet parallel and heels approximately 6 inches away from the wall. Bend your knees so that your buttocks are lowered 4 or 5 inches. Keeping your tail against the wall let your trunk, head and arms curl forwards in a relaxed manner. Now gradually uncurl your spine against the wall, pressing each vertebra in turn against it until your spine is fully in contact with the wall. Pause and then repeat 3 times more.

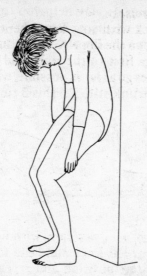

Strengthening Exercises

1. Lying on your back, with the knees bent and the soles of
   the feet resting on the floor, hands by your sides, raise
   your head to look at your knees, and tighten the
   abdominal muscles. Hold for a count of 3, relax and
   repeat twice.

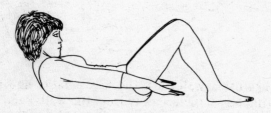

2. Stand with your back against a wall and place your feet
   about 6 inches apart so that your heels are 10 inches or
   so away from the wall. Let your knees bend so that your
   buttocks slide about 10 inches down the wall and hold
   for a count of 10. Straighten up and relax before repeating

a further 4 times. It may help you to have your hands resting on your thighs, or alternatively to hold on to a chair, placed at one side of you for support.

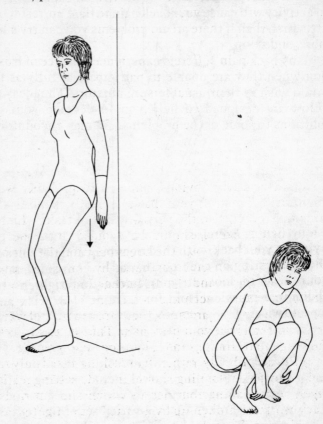

3. Stand with your feet parallel and about 8 inches apart. Now squat down slowly, keeping your heels on the ground, until your thighs touch your calf muscles. Hold this position for a count of 5 before straightening up slowly and then repeat a further 4 times. You may either let your arms hang freely at your side or alternatively put them on your thighs as you lower and raise.

Avoiding Back Pain in Leisure Activities

By this stage you should be fit enough to contemplate other forms of general exercise. If you are in doubt about whether an activity will cause your back pain to flare up, test it out a little first, then if there are no problems you can try a little more, and so on.

Many back pain sufferers experience a degree of frustration when they are unable to participate as fully as they would wish in their usual leisure pursuits. The ideas that follow are designed to help you to develop your own solutions to some of the problems you may encounter.

Gardening

It should be fairly obvious, but is still probably worth emphasizing, that if your back is really painful then gardening, other than the very gentlest of tasks which do not involve bending, should be avoided until the pain begins to resolve. Those who are prone to recurrent back pain will know to their cost how little it takes to provoke the onset of pain, and the price that has to be paid for persistent or heavy activity.

If you enjoy your gardening there are a variety of ways in which you can beat your back pain. The key to survival is knowing your limits, and planning and grading your activities accordingly, rather than rushing ahead only to be stopped by pain. Planning should include setting realistic targets, establishing routines in which short periods of heavy work are broken up by a varied set of lighter tasks, and choosing the tools to help you minimize stress.

Stooping and bending tend to cause a lot of trouble, and this can be avoided by using long-handled tools and by kneeling down rather than stooping with a bent back: a number of kneelers are available on the market for those who experience difficulty in getting into a kneeling position. When cutting the lawn or hedge, it is important not to try to do too much at one time and to avoid reaching above head height. It might well be an idea to consider purchasing a mechanized mower and hedge-cutter, although you will need to bear in mind their weight.

Handling heavy weights, as when digging, can also easily cause back pain, so do read the guidelines on lifting in Chapter 4 and apply them here. If you absolutely must dig your garden, it may be wise to invest in a spade and fork that provide mechanical assistance. At the least, you should make sure you use a good-quality spade and only dig a moderate spadeful each time.

Above all else, it is vital to get used to the idea of doing a little at a time, and if your back pain is of the type that is likely to be of long duration you might even do well to consider changing the format of your garden. Raised beds, herbaceous borders and simple lawns can do much to take the backache out of gardening.

Sports

As more people participate in sporting activities it is inevitable that the incidence of back pain will increase. Although sometimes injury is unavoidable, usually back injuries are the result of poor technique, inadequate preparation and lack of fitness. Those who do sustain back injuries while playing sports should seek prompt treatment and learn how to avoid further trouble. On no account should they resume participation until they are fully fit again.

The sports that are especially suitable for those with back pain are ones in which free and rhythmic movements are a major feature. Walking and gentle running on grass, swimming and cycling, all tend to be well tolerated. However, most other sports can be undertaken as long as the advice and guidance of a competent coach have been sought first. Proficiency, care and fitness are the only ways to avoid further injury.

Ultimately, no one but you will be able to judge whether a particular sport aggravates your back problem. As a general rule, always try out any new activity for a short time before going into it flat out. When in doubt, seek the advice of experts.

Backs and Sex

It is not uncommon for those who suffer with back pain, or who have undergone a spinal operation, to have some initial difficulty with sexual intercourse. In some instances acute pain – or even the fear of pain – can result in the affected partner's appearing to become somewhat physically distant, tense, or frigid. This sort of situation can be an added worry at an already difficult time.

During the early painful period following an attack of back pain or immediately after a spinal operation, sexual activity should be approached with caution. As healing and recovery take place, sexual relations can gradually be resumed as long as it is agreed by both partners that activities must be discontinued if there is any major increase in pain. During the return to normality there will almost certainly be occasions when problems will occur and frustration may result. However, with understanding, total frankness and a great deal of kindness there is no reason why normal sexual relationships should not be possible in a matter of a few weeks.

There will always be a small percentage of back pain sufferers who will find sexual activity uncomfortable and even unpleasant. This may be due to chronic degenerative changes in the spinal system or additionally, in women, may be associated with a gynaecological problem. Should you fall into this category, do talk to your doctor or therapist who may be able to advise you or put you in contact with a counsellor who specializes in sexual problems related to physical disability. There are also a number of excellent books on human sexuality.

It is well worth exploring the subject in some depth to discover the variety of techniques and positions that exist. Some of the ideas you come across may seem outside the bounds of your current experience, but it is a mistake to think that there is something abnormal or even deviant about trying new positions. Essentially, any position that enables both partners to share pleasure in each other is not going to be harmful, and can play a beneficial part in moving towards a full and normal lifestyle after back injury.

8 *Seeking Medical Help*

The idea of helping and caring for oneself is admirable and to be encouraged, but some kinds of back pain require the attention of medically qualified experts who specialize in the treatment of the spine and all its complications. Of the 23 million episodes of back pain that are estimated to occur every year in the United Kingdom, many must resolve fairly quickly, but about 3 million initial visits are nevertheless made to family doctors in the same period. Out of these 3 million a small minority, some 33,000 patients, have to be referred for consultant advice.

The Family Doctor

Most people who have back pain see their family doctor for advice and treatment, and for many this is all that is necessary. One point that needs to be appreciated is that your doctor has chosen to be a 'general practitioner' and therefore has to have a very broad range of experience in order to cover all patients from the newborn to the terminally ill. It is self-evident that it is not possible for the GP to have the depth of knowledge of a specialist on all aspects of medical care. Your doctor's specialized interests are likely to reflect hospital placements as a junior houseman or a particular interest that has subsequently developed. Usually in a group practice the doctors cover certain areas as their specialities. If your doctor is interested in back problems then you will probably receive a good deal of help, but if his or her main interests are in other areas then you may obtain only a basic level of treatment.

The most important thing your doctor should do for you is to make as accurate a diagnosis as possible, and in particular to identify if the symptoms are sufficiently serious to warrant a specialist's opinion. Although a definite diagnosis is not always easy to achieve in a busy overworked surgery, it should be possible to obtain a reasonable history of your problem and then undertake a clinical examination which will provide a fairly clear picture. Most patients with back pain do not require blood tests or X-ray investigation, though these options are available if they are considered necessary.

The treatment that you may expect to receive at this stage will be basic, and usually consists of advice to rest and some form of analgesia and/or muscle-relaxant tablets to ease spasm and reduce pain. Interestingly, a study of the choice of medicines for low back pain revealed that aspirin was still one of the most successful medications available. The gastric side-effects associated with aspirin may be eliminated by the use of micro-encapsulation or enteric-coated tablets.

Should your doctor decide that your problem is mechanical or inflammatory in origin and requires more specialized attention, you could be sent to a consultant specialist. Alternatively, if your local hospital physiotherapy department accepts referrals from general practitioners (this is called 'direct GP access'), you may be referred directly for physiotherapy without first going to a consultant. As a third possibility, if you wish you could be referred to a private physiotherapist or occasionally even to a complementary practitioner. Some doctors who have undergone specialist training in manipulative therapy or acupuncture techniques are able to provide these forms of treatment themselves.

It is easy to underrate the importance of the family doctor in the treatment chain for spinal problems. Your GP has to accept a great deal of responsibility in the initial stages, and even after referral to hospital will be responsible to a certain extent for your aftercare. There is a growing trend towards early treatment, and in the majority of mechanical lesions the use of manipulation, massage, spinal supports and graded exercise can result in a speedy recovery.

The Hospital Consultant

When a general practitioner is uncertain of the cause of a patient's back pain or considers the problem to be sufficiently serious to warrant a second opinion, the patient will be referred to a consultant specialist, usually in a large general hospital.

The choice of the consultant you see in the first instance will depend on the nature of your complaint and the contacts your family doctor has established. If your condition is serious there will probably be no delay before seeing a specialist, but if the problem is considered to be less urgent you may have to wait a number of weeks for an appointment in the National Health Service. The only alternative is to see a consultant privately and pay the fees yourself or through a medical insurance scheme.

Orthopaedic surgeon. Up to 70 per cent of patients with back pain will be referred to an orthopaedic surgeon, who specializes in the musculo-skeletal system. Within this group there are a growing number who specialize particularly in spinal problems.

Neurosurgeon. A smaller number of back sufferers are referred to a consultant neurosurgeon, whose expertise is related primarily to the central and peripheral nervous system.

Neurologist. The neurologist's speciality is similar to that of the neurosurgeon, except that the neurologist is a physician and this approach does not involve surgery. Patients who are referred to a neurologist usually have a problem which is not easily identifiable and requires extensive careful investigation.

Rheumatologist. Consultants in rheumatology and rehabilitation deal with inflammatory problems related to the soft tissues as well as with various forms of arthritis. The treatment provided by this group is conservative, but if necessary you may be referred to a surgeon. Treatments may include anti-inflammatory drug therapy, injections and physiotherapy. Your doctor will send you to a rheumatologist if it is suspected that your problem is inflammatory rather than mechanical in origin, and here again there are rheumatologists who specialize in back care and have a great deal of expertise.

Consultant anaesthetist. Some of these organize pain clinics, special centres for those patients with chronic intractable pain which has not responded to other forms of treatment. Pain clinics are non-surgical in their approach and are often used when other measures have been unsuccessful.

Psychiatrist. Only a small percentage of back pain sufferers see a psychiatrist. Unfortunately, many consider it a personal insult to visit a psychiatrist for a complaint of this kind, presumably because of the implication that their pain is imagined. This is far from the truth. As was suggested earlier, back pain is a complex physical and psychological mixture. Both aspects of the pain are very real and significant from the point of view of the sufferer. The psychiatrist specializes in the resolution of the psychological components of back pain and is an invaluable member of the team, whose expertise lies in identifying underlying problems related to tension and stress and in providing methods of relief and relaxation. Psychiatric referral therefore should be viewed as just another way of exploring relevant aspects of your back pain.

The various consultants within this group do not work in isolation, recognizing their own limitations as well as those of their colleagues. It is quite common for patients to see more than one specialist, and it is one of the strengths of the National Health Service that access to this wealth of expertise is the automatic right of all patients.

Investigations for Back Pain

The successful treatment of back pain depends on an accurate identification of the cause, and on finding an appropriate response in order to resolve it. The first and most important investigation involves taking your personal account of the problem. This is followed by a clinical examination which may last anything from fifteen minutes to an hour. On the basis of the personal history and the doctor's findings it is usually possible to identify, in broad terms, the primary source of the trouble.

Most patients seen by hospital consultants have at least a simple X-ray taken, but in those cases where surgery or some other form of internal treatment is envisaged more complicated measures will be necessary, involving the use of radio-opaque dyes. On occasions laboratory tests will be made on blood and tissue samples in an attempt to identify if there is evidence of infection or inflammatory changes. It is better, as a general rule, to over-investigate and thus eliminate all possible causes of pain than to under-investigate and miss some small yet important clue.

Personal History

This is an essential investigation designed to uncover all the relevant details about your lifestyle and general health and how these relate to your back problems past and present. The kinds of questions you may be asked are shown in the self-assessment questionnaire that appears in Chapter 3. The chief skill required of the questioner is to make patients relax and to guide them carefully in a structured way into giving a full and clear picture of what has happened and how the pain affects them. Possibly because they have been overawed by the occasion, patients may find afterwards that they have forgotten to mention some vital point which has concerned them. A useful trick is to write down in advance your key points, which you can check before you finally leave the consulting room. Listen carefully to the questions before responding. The best results come from answers that are clear, to the point, and fairly brief. If the consultant requires more detail you are sure to be asked for it.

The Clinical Examination

This examination will be carried out only by a consultant, a doctor or a physiotherapist: it is important to try to relax because otherwise tension may cloud the real symptoms. Your examination begins as soon as you walk into the consulting room, and the examiner will be watching the way you walk, sit, stand and hold yourself. The exact nature of the examination may vary according to the individual conducting it, but usually you will be observed while standing, before your spinal movements are checked for limitations in bending, straightening and turning. After this you will probably be asked to sit on the edge of a couch whilst your knee reflexes are tested. Various passive movements may also be carried out to discover limitations of range or their effect upon the pain. From now on all the tests are done to target the exact source of your pain.

It is normal next to be asked to lie on your back, and in this position the strength of various muscle groups will be tested, as well as the height to which you can raise your leg when it is held straight. Skin sensation may also be checked at this stage. Finally you will be asked to lie flat, face downwards, and after the normal tests for muscle strength and sensation have been done, the most important part of your examination will occur. Your spine will be palpated from the base of your skull to the coccyx, and each vertebral segment will be felt for any bony abnormalities, muscle tension, areas of tenderness or other physical signs. Usually you will unconsciously indicate areas of pain by muscle spasm in an attempt to guard your injury, and the skilled examiner will check with you at all times to see which areas are especially tender.

X-Ray

The plain, standard X-ray films of the spine are taken in most cases of low back pain referred to a consultant, and can reveal the more obvious causes. Joint displacement, crush fractures, infective lesions and chemical changes due to the ageing process are usually easy to pinpoint. However, the identification of soft tissue lesions in the spinal system involves more detailed studies using radio-opaque contrast media, which outline the areas around the discs and nerve roots. Of these, the myelogram and the discogram are two of the techniques used and will serve as examples of this kind of procedure.

Myelogram

This investigation is normally undertaken when there are strong indications of a ruptured intervertebral disc which is likely to require surgery. Myelography may be used in cases where there is a long history of back pain, possibly with indications of nerve-root entrapment, which has failed to respond to any other treatment. The investigation involves the insertion of a special hollow needle very carefully into the area of the lesions, through which a contrast medium is introduced. This mixes with the cerebro-spinal fluid, permitting the soft structures around the spinal cord and nerve roots to become visible on the X-ray. A series of pictures is taken and then the dye is withdrawn as is the lumbar puncture needle. Although it is natural to feel apprehensive about this type of procedure, it may reassure you to know that it has been done many times on thousands of patients and very rarely causes more than some minor discomfort.

Discogram

This technique is used to examine the intervertebral discs. As it is likely to be more painful, patients are given some mild sedation in order to make the procedure more comfortable. As with the myelogram, a lumbar puncture needle is first introduced into the disc spaces to be examined and through this the contrast medium is injected directly into the discs. X-ray pictures are taken immediately and sometimes also after an interval of 15 – 20 minutes.

As before, the lumbar puncture needle is removed at the conclusion of the X-rays. Whilst this procedure may be slightly painful, it is the only available technique which can provide the consultant with a clear picture of exactly what is happening to a disc.

Computerized Tomography (CAT Scans)

Most people become aware of CAT scanners as a result of appeals launched for their purchase. As each machine can cost over a million pounds, it is highly unlikely that any but the major teaching hospitals would have such equipment, but for public generosity. The main advantage of CAT scanners is that they permit a very accurate examination of the body without the necessity to introduce needles or radio-opaque dye. In addition, unlike normal X-rays, a CAT scan is able to show up soft tissues as well as bone and tissues enclosed within bone. The pictures provided by CAT scanners are, in effect, sliver-thin slices through the area under examination and the full scope of these machines and other more advanced models that have been introduced recently has yet to be exploited. One thing is certain, it will make the process of diagnosis much more accurate, simple, painless and safe for the patient.

Diagnostic Ultrasound

Developed at the Doncaster Royal Infirmary by Mr Richard Porter, a consultant orthopaedic surgeon, this technique, which is non-invasive and does not involve the use of needles or radio-opaque dye, is used to measure the diameter of the spinal canal. It is an extremely safe method of examining the spine and is totally without any pain. Although Richard Porter's team has mastered the technique and made it into a simple routine investigation, it has yet to be adopted in other centres.

Laboratory Tests

Blood tests are sometimes used as a back-up screening process for patients who have severe back pain, particularly in the elderly, where metabolic disorders are suspected. The most common tests used include complete blood count, E.S.R. (the rate of sedimentation of red cells, which indicates the presence of an inflammatory state) and other blood tests for calcium, phosphate and alkaline phosphates.

In the cases where inflammatory back pain is suspected, blood tests are vital and the only positive method of identification.

Surgery for Back Pain

The chances that you will have to have surgery are fairly small, something like one in 2,500. If you are referred to hospital the odds shorten to one in 350. The likelihood of surgery will be indicated by the cause of your pain.

The use of surgery to resolve back pain is a final resort and rarely selected unless there are positive signs of serious nerve root or spinal cord involvement. For the vast majority of sufferers conservative measures are very successful. Chemonucleolysis, the chemical dissolving of disc protrusions, is a relatively recent innovation, which may lead to a dramatic reduction in the need for surgical intervention. At present there are some twenty centres in the United Kingdom where this technique has been adopted as a routine measure.

The success rate of spinal surgery is fairly high, though a small percentage of those who undergo a spinal operation will experience varying degrees of post-operative discomfort. This is probably due to the body's reaction to the disturbance of the spinal tissues, but there are some new forms of electrotherapy which can improve post-operative healing rates and help to reduce the pain and swelling that may result from surgery.

Spinal surgery is only considered after extensive investigation, where there is persistent deep-seated pain, progressive numbness or muscle weakness or loss of bowel and bladder control. In virtually every instance the causative agent will be mechanical, for example the contents of the disc will have ruptured and be pressing on the nerve root or the spinal cord. Alternatively, the nerve root may be restricted by bony outgrowths from the facet joint, or the spinal cord may have become compressed by a narrowed spinal canal. When there is a significant degree of segmental instability, which permits an abnormal amount of movement between adjacent vertebrae, surgical fixation may be the only solution.

Except in this last instance, the main aim of spinal surgery is to remove any obstructions that may be pressing on the nerve root and spinal cord in order to free these structures. The operations in this category include laminectomy for the removal of protruded disc material or a damaged disc, and facetectomy in which a portion of the facet joint is trimmed off to remove pressure from the nerve root. When the spinal cord or nerve root is trapped or constricted, the operation may be called a spinal decompression.

As the operation called laminectomy is one of the most common techniques used to gain access to the spinal column, a brief description of it will be given here. Spinal fusion will also be considered, as an example of another common spinal operation.

Laminectomy

The usual site for a laminectomy is over the three lower spinal vertebrae and the sacrum. The incision is normally longitudinal, though some surgeons prefer a transverse approach.

After the tissues of the spine have been eased away from the bony structures on the side of the spine where the problem is located, a small 'window' is created by nibbling away part or all of the bony arch covering the spinal cord and nerve root. The tissues overlying the nerve root and cord are then moved gently to one side, and the extruded disc material is removed. Often the interior of the disc is also cleaned as there is always the chance that the disc could otherwise cause further trouble. When there is any disc material adhering to the nerve root this is removed prior to closing up the wound.

Spinal Fusion

In those instances when one or more segments of the spinal column become unstable due to wear and tear, or following the removal of an intervertebral disc that has been damaged so severely it cannot be saved, the surgeon will have to fuse the vertebrae together. Fusion is normally achieved using bone grafts over the facets and the neural arch (which covers the spinal canal) at the back of the vertebrae, or alternatively some surgeons prefer to fuse the bodies of the vertebrae together. Wires or clamps may be used to ensure stability whilst the required bony fusion takes place.

The post-operative routine will initially be slower than that for most other spinal operations. However, once there are signs that the bone graft has been successful, then great stress will be placed on your regaining spinal movements and returning to a normal lifestyle.

Post-Operative Routines

These will vary from centre to centre, but the regime described here is a typical example of what might follow a spinal operation.

On your return from the operating theatre you are likely to be laid flat on your back for the first four hours and then assisted to turn on to one side, your back, and the other side at two-hourly intervals to prevent the development of pressure sores. On the day after your operation you will be encouraged to move, and will probably stand for a short time. Should you experience difficulty in using a bed pan or urinal, you may be permitted a short walk to the toilet. By the next day you can expect to be sitting out of bed, and walking a few steps every two hours or so. If your progress has been satisfactory you could begin some spinal bending exercises under the strict guidance of your physiotherapist. On the third post-operative day you should be able to move around at will, though it would be wise to adopt a policy of 'little and often'. If you listen to your body it will tell you when it is ready to progress. Your stitches will normally be removed at the end of the first week, at which point you can expect to go home, possibly wearing a simple spinal support.

Once at home you will be expected gradually to increase the amount you do each day, including some specific spinal exercises along the lines of the routines described earlier. A fortnight after the operation you can go for a short car journey, but it will be a further three weeks before you can consider driving yourself. If your job is a fairly light office one, you will be able to return to work four to six weeks after your operation. If, however, it involves heavy physical activity, then your return will have to be delayed for up to three months.

Once your body begins to recover from the operation it is important to get yourself back to a reasonable level of general fitness by progressive use of exercise. After six weeks you should be able to undertake most normal tasks – though it is vital to remember to use your spine properly in the way you have been taught by your physiotherapist – and at the end of four months you may consider yourself fully back to normal and able to forget that you ever had a back injury. The progress that you make will depend largely on yourself. If ever in doubt about anything to do with your operation, ask your doctor or the consultant who performed the operation.

Chemonucleolysis

The term chemonucleolysis is used to describe the chemical dissolution of disc material which is causing back pain by pressing on nerve roots or the spinal cord. The chemical used for this purpose is chymopapain, which is a naturally occurring enzyme found in the papaya tree.

The first trials were made on chymopapain in 1963, and although there were initial claims of a 70 per cent success rate chymopapain was taken off the American market in 1975, because of unsatisfactory side-effects, and has only recently been reintroduced in a refined form. The results are constantly under review.

The technique used to introduce the chemical is similar to that used for a discogram described earlier. It is injected directly into the nuclear material of the disc and immediately starts to break down certain tissue bands within the damaged nucleus, converting it into a soft slush. Initially there will be a rise in the disc pressure, which may cause a marginal increase in pain, but this settles down rapidly, within a few hours. Over a period of two or three weeks the extruded nuclear material shrinks under the action of the chymopapain and the pressure on the nerve root is reduced, as is the associated pain. It is believed this process continues for a further two months. There is some research evidence to suggest that discs injected with chymopapain gradually return to a near-normal healthy state.

As yet the use of chemonucleolysis is still in a developmental stage, and whilst the indications are very encouraging the technique should not be seen as a miracle cure. This new breakthrough in the treatment of back pain due to disc rupture will need a great deal more careful testing to determine exactly which patients are likely to derive most benefit from the proper use of chymopapain and how the technique can be formalized to take its place as a routine alternative to spinal surgery.

9 *Further Help for Back Pain*

Physiotherapy Services

The vast majority of patients who are referred to a hospital consultant with back pain will be treated at some time by a physiotherapist, though the actual techniques will vary to some extent from place to place and therapist to therapist.

Now that the rules of professional conduct have been modified to permit physiotherapists to act as independent practitioners, taking on patients directly, without referral, treatment and advice should become more readily available and at an earlier stage. Physiotherapists in private practice also offer an early opportunity for patients to receive treatment.

With the increase in knowledge about back problems, physiotherapists have been moving away from a reliance mainly on the use of heat massage and exercises in favour of a more broadly based scheme. This reflects a growing awareness of the need for back pain patients to be considered in a more comprehensive way on the basis of all their symptoms and circumstances. Various hospitals have pioneered systems of back care and back fitness designed for chronic back pain patients who have failed to find relief from any other form of treatment.

These programmes have been developed to meet the varied needs of individual patients, and recognize that, given the complexity of back pain syndrome, no single measure is likely to be totally successful. Instead, a combination of naturally based therapeutic measures is employed to help the body to heal itself. These include the use of heat, cold, light, ultrasound, vibration, and manual and mechanical measures including friction and manipulation, hydrotherapy and exercise. Some elements of these originate in the medical practices of the ancient Chinese, Indians, Arabs and Greeks.

A typical back care programme is likely to have some of the following components:

- Clinical examination.
- Patient-administered subjective evaluation.
- Functional assessment.
- Individual treatments as appropriate.
- Back school.
- Follow-up and support.
- Evaluation.

Clinical Examination

Although nearly all the patients who are seen by physiotherapists will have been examined and diagnosed by a GP, and possibly also by a consultant, it is normal practice for a physiotherapist to undertake a further, detailed examination including history and physical examination. This is necessary in order to make sure that the case is fully assessed in the light of the treatment that can be provided. Existing medical records will have been consulted beforehand, and X-ray and blood test results checked.

Patient-Administered Subjective Evaluation (P.A.S.E.)

This is a structured questionnaire which is given to the patient to complete, and resembles the questionnaire detailed in Chapter 3. There is a distinct possibility that in the course of the clinical examination patients may not manage to say all that they themselves wished. The P.A.S.E. is designed to fill this vital gap and to let back pain sufferers really express their feelings, guided by the questions that are on the form. At the completion of the treatment the form may again be useful to demonstrate to the patient the degree of progress that has been made.

Functional Assessments

These are used to establish the level of functional disability that is present. The patient is asked to perform a series of daily activities and is scored on performance and for the time taken. Observations are made on the way the individual sits, stands, gets into and out of bed, climbs stairs, walks a 440-yard circuit, washes up and packs shopping. The activities can be varied to reflect the person's lifestyle. (In the U.S.A. this type of evaluation is replaced by a special form of obstacle course.) Because the judgment of the therapist undertaking the assessment is inevitably subjective, the scoring system has to be carefully structured to eliminate any bias, and is checked by another therapist from time to time. Should a patient's performance indicate that there are serious difficulties related to home or work activities, then corrective action will need to be taken as a matter of urgency.

Appropriate Treatment

Following the initial clinical assessment, and before any patient can be considered for the later stages of rehabilitation, it is important to deal with the immediate back pain if this is at all possible. To this end a variety of the techniques already mentioned may be used, either in combination or as isolated measures, and might also include the provision of a suitable spinal support.

Back School

The idea of the back school was originally conceived by a Swedish physiotherapist, Marianne Zacrisson Forsell, in 1969. Observing the limited success of the routine physiotherapeutic attempts to resolve back pain, she decided that the time had come to adopt a more radical approach using exercise, ergonomics and education to inform patients about their condition, to enable them to gain a reasonable degree of fitness, and to modify their activities sensibly at home and work. The hoped-for goal was to restore normality and prevent relapse. The back school system was a success, and soon the idea was taken up in North America and Australia; it was first tried in the United Kingdom in 1975. At present there are at least fifty back schools within the

National Health Service and private back schools are just being formed.

The length of time spent in a back school can vary considerably from centre to centre, but attendance every weekday for a fortnight is probably the optimum required to rehabilitate patients without making too-heavy demands on their work time or domestic arrangements. During this period, Mondays, Wednesdays and Fridays might be spent on health education exercises and practical advice on proper use of the body, with Tuesdays and Thursdays devoted to relaxation and the restoration of mobility in a hydrotherapy pool. The use of a hydrotherapy pool, which is maintained at a temperature of around 94°F, is a valuable part of the whole programme. The warmth and buoyancy of the pool can achieve amazing results in just a few treatment sessions.

The exercise and relaxation routines that are used in back schools are similar to those found in the earlier chapters of this book. Some back schools use slide-tape programmes, and others make video films of patients at the beginning and end of treatment in order to see the results of treatment and education. Yet others prefer to rely on the teaching and guidance provided by a team of experienced physiotherapists who specialize in back care. Interplay between the individual patients and the therapist permits the progress of each class to be tailored and modified to meet the particular needs of the group.

At the end of the programme it is usual to spend some time in the gymnasium, where the lessons learnt about the body and how it functions are applied to a number of daily activities, especially the moving and lifting of heavy objects. The aim is not so much to make the group proficient in handling particular loads, but instead to encourage individuals to think about various typical tasks and then to find the best solution based on their new-found understanding of themselves and their backs. This includes learning the art of knowing one's personal limitations, and avoiding those things which might cause symptoms to flare up again. Although this may sound idealistic, the result is that less than 15 per cent of patients are likely to need to return for further treatment.

Follow-Up Support

A few patients who have chronic back problems may never recover and do require some degree of continuing support. People in this category may be invited to attend for a hydrotherapy pool session every week, if they feel the need. This can prove very helpful, as such a session provides not only physical therapy but group support. In one or two back schools patients are given an individually tailored exercise circuit which they can perform as part of a hospital-based back group, and at home.

Evaluation

All patients who have completed a programme of therapy and education should, ideally, be reviewed every six months to check on their progress. Unfortunately, however, the resources of the hospital services do not at present permit this.

Spinal Supports

There is no reason to suppose that even our early ancestors did not use some form of binding to support their backs when they hurt – the earliest known support, made of birch bark and dated around 900 AD, is to be found in the Colorado State Hospital Museum, U.S.A. – and the use of a good spinal support remains a helpful adjunct to any system of back care.

Spinal supports in Europe can be traced back to before the twelfth century, but the steel and fabric supports, which have only recently been improved on, almost certainly owe their origins to the fashion corsetry which was in vogue from the sixteenth to the nineteenth centuries. Over the past decade, these steel and fabric supports have been steadily declining in popularity with the introduction of more comfortable but effective supports made from elasticated fabric and thermoplastic pads. The statistics suggest that spinal supports are still a popular form of therapy, and up to 70 per cent of those seeing a hospital consultant are likely to be issued with some form of support.

At one time it was believed that the purpose of a spinal support was to restrict the movement in the lower spine and thereby limit pain. However, research conducted in the mid-1960s disproved this concept, and it has now been discovered that the modern elasticated lumbo-sacral support enhances intra-abdominal pressure and provides natural splintage for the spine. Additionally, the support pad retains body heat and keeps the area warm. This, and the associated pressure of the pad against the painful area, helps to reduce muscle spasm and the accompanying pain.

Most people with back pain experience a loss of confidence at the onset of their attack, and the vast majority of patients who have been provided with a modern lumbo-sacral support have been surprised at the confidence it gives them and also at how comfortable and natural it feels. The range of pain-free spinal movement is increased whilst at the same time the support acts as a reminder of the need for proper respect for, and use of, the spinal system.

Three types of lumbo-sacral support are commonly provided:

1. An elasticated support with a rigid thermoplastic pad which is heat-moulded to fit the contours of the patient's back. This is primarily used for the relatively small number of patients who may have a nerve entrapment or some other mechanical problem in which spinal movements need to be limited for a short period.
2. A slightly longer elasticated support with a plastic foam pad at the front and rear. This is generally used, after an initial period of bed rest, for patients who have a very acute back problem. It is also sometimes used for patients who have major degenerative changes in their spine. The support provides firm bracing for the spine

and abdomen and tends to restrict movement in the lower lumbar spine, enabling patients to rapidly regain a more mobile state, and in some instances to return to light work within a matter of days.

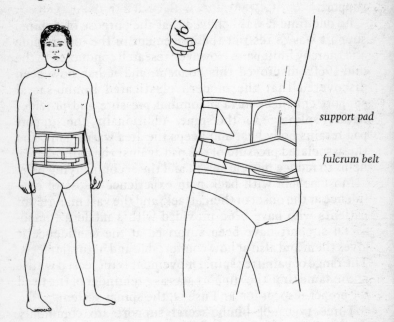

support pad

fulcrum belt

A modern lumbo-sacral support

3. A lightweight lumbo-sacral support with only a pad at the back, which is probably the most regularly prescribed. This is designed to be worn during the sub-acute and recovery stage. Because it gives support, increases confidence and encourages movement, it is an invaluable complement to the progressive rehabilitation of back pain patients.

As a matter of policy, no spinal support should ever be issued without a prior examination. Supports are intended for short-term use during the acute, sub-acute and early stages of final recovery, and all patients should be taught a series of exercises to enable them gradually to dispense with the support over a period of weeks. However, those who have a residual disability are advised to use their supports whenever they plan to undertake stressful activity which is likely to aggravate their back pain, in order to help reduce the strain on the spine. In some cases also, back pain sufferers are provided with a support for use at work.

Overall, in the context of an active treatment programme, spinal supports have a vital role to play, particularly in the early restoration of mobility and confidence.

Pain Clinics

Modern medical science has made many advances in the resolution of disease and injury processes but it has to be admitted that, although this does not include the majority of back pain cases, there remain conditions with associated intractable pain which have not yet been mastered. One of the commonest causes of deep-seated, long-term pain is musculo-skeletal disease, particularly that affecting the back, and according to some estimates this underlies as many as 50 per cent of all referrals to pain clinics.

Patients are normally referred to a pain clinic by their family doctor, consultant orthopaedic surgeon or physician, and by the time they are referred many may already have had extensive treatment, including surgery. Before any further treatment can be embarked on, however, it will be necessary again for the past clinical history to be reviewed including the checking of hospital notes, X-rays, laboratory tests, and psychiatric reports if these exist. This will then be followed by a very careful physical examination in order to determine the cause, or at least the site, of pain and to establish a firm diagnosis.

Because of the very nature of the problems seen in the pain clinic, there can be no definitive regime which can be used in every case. The whole aim of the pain clinic is to provide a centre where a variety of techniques can be utilized, in order to discover the particular method, or combination of methods, that is best suited to the needs of the patient. Treatments commonly used include anti-inflammatory drugs, anti-depressant therapy, on occasions psychological counselling, muscle-relaxant drugs, pain-relieving injections and certain forms of physiotherapy. In some cases acupuncture may be tried, and very occasionally hypnotherapy.

The function of anti-inflammatory drugs, judicious anti-depressant therapy and muscle relaxants should be fairly obvious and there is no need to discuss them further here.

Pain-Relieving Injections

At the simplest level these can take the form of infiltration of local anaesthetic into painful 'trigger points', into supra-spinous and interspinous ligaments of the spine, and into the facet joints' nerve supply. In those cases where the patterns of pain follow the distribution of an identifiable nerve root or roots, the pain may be relieved by an injection around the painful areas or into the space around the irritated nerve root. It may be necessary to repeat the procedure three or four times over a six-week period before full pain relief can be achieved.

When the pain is severe and persistent it may become necessary to destroy the nerve, either by the injection of a chemical agent, or surgical division, but this is normally considered as a last resort.

Electrical Pain Control Procedures

The control of pain by electrical means is a fairly new innovation introduced into Britain after the technique had been proved successful in the U.S.A. Surprisingly, the earliest records of this form of pain relief appear in the descriptions of Hippocratic medicine around 6 BC. It seems that a Greek named Anteros, who had gout, stepped on an electric torpedo fish which was hidden in shallow sea water where Anteros was paddling, presumably to ease his gout. The fish, who resented being trodden on, gave Anteros a nasty 30 – 40 volt shock. After hopping around, Anteros discovered his foot didn't hurt any more, and this is said to be the way this form of therapy started.

The modern equivalent of the torpedo fish is a small battery-powered generator, often not much bigger than a match box. This is called a Transcutaneous Electronic Nerve Stimulator, or TENS. The apparatus is used to transmit low-powered electrical stimuli across the surface of the skin to the nervous system by means of small

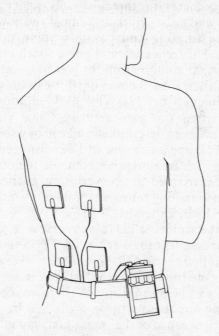

TENS in position on the back

electrodes attached to the skin and connected to the TENS equipment. No one is absolutely certain how TENS works, but it is known to block the transmission of pain signals to the pain centres of the brain, possibly by interfering with the normal pain mechanisms. Before you can be issued with a TENS, a careful examination is necessary to determine the areas and levels of your pain. Most doctors and therapists who use TENS apparatus will place the small 'rubber' electrodes over a number of sites until they find the location which gives the greatest relief. In some instances the electrodes are placed along traditional acupuncture lines, or alternatively, spanning a painful trigger point.

Once the electrodes are in place and connected to the TENS, the doctor or therapist will select a particular frequency and pulse-width and adjust the power until you experience tingling and possibly some minor muscle twitching. The frequency and pulse-width may be altered until the right combination for you has been found. The current is then turned down until it can only just be felt. Each treatment usually lasts for 30–45 minutes and is then repeated when the pain returns. Once your personal settings have been determined and you have been taught to use the TENS apparatus you will be permitted to continue with your own treatment at home. It is not unusual for TENS to be provided on a prescription, in the same way as the person with long-term pain problems would use powerful analgesic drug therapy.

One of the secrets of TENS is to persevere, as it may take a while for an effect to be achieved. TENS should never be used when there is no pain, and there is every chance that the effects of stimulation will last longer and longer until the TENS can be discontinued. There are certain contra-indications but these will be explained by whoever fits your TENS. Because of the individual way in which TENS has to be applied, the practice of sending people to the local supplier to be issued with a TENS without proper instruction is ill-advised.

The advantages of TENS are its effectiveness, that it is not a drug-based therapy, and that it can be used at any time by anyone of average intelligence. It is very compact and designed to be unobtrusive under normal clothes. Last, but not least, TENS is a relatively inexpensive way of controlling persistent pain. It does not always work with back pain, but if it is ineffective make sure this is not due to lack of perseverance or to incorrect fitting.

Acupuncture

Acupuncture has featured as part of Chinese medical practice since before the year 210 BC. At that time sharpened stones were used to prick certain sites on the body for the relief of pain. Gradually the sharpened stones were replaced with fine needles made of bone and bamboo and later these

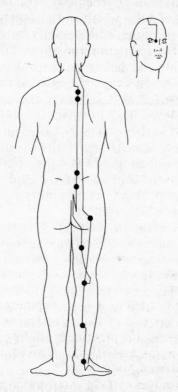

A typical acupuncture meridian used for back pain

were discarded in favour of the steel, silver and gold needles used in modern acupuncture techniques. In the traditional Chinese medical philosophy the life force has two equal and opposite forces, the 'yin' and the 'yang'. When people are in a healthy state the yin and yang forces are in a settled and balanced state, but should there be any disharmony and imbalance between these two elements sickness and disease will result. The Chinese have identified twelve main channels along which the yin and yang life forces flow and on these channels there are over 700 separate points which can be stimulated in order to restore the yin-yang balance.

In traditional acupuncture the acupuncture points are stimulated by inserting the special needles to a particular depth and then gently rotating them. This produces a deep aching feeling and also often reduces the initial pain. On some occasions heat may be applied to the acupuncture needles, or used by itself over the acupuncture point. Heating is produced by placing and lighting a small pyramid of a herbal substance called moxa over the point. The patient is asked to report when heating is experienced, and the smouldering moxa is then removed. In Western medicine some acupuncturists apply small electrical currents to the acupuncture points via the needles, after these have been inserted.

Although Western medical practitioners increasingly accept that acupuncture techniques have a pain-relieving effect in a number of cases, not all accept the theories about the yin and yang life forces. Studies have revealed that in most instances the Chinese acupuncture points relate very closely to so-called trigger points. In about 70 per cent of cases the patterns of pain associated with trigger and acupuncture points are very similar. It is likely that sedation of painful tissues by means of acupuncture, or the Japanese acupressure, or by transcutaneous electronic nerve stimulation, all successfully operate by inhibiting pain. The sites of activity are possibly in the brain stem.

There seems to be no doubt that acupuncture, when applied by a properly trained practitioner, may be able to relieve pain in the back and its associated misery. Schools and colleges of acupuncture exist in Britain and a number of doctors have undertaken some form of training. If you decide to visit an acupuncturist on your own initiative, however, it would be wise to find out what his or her local reputation is like, as there is no standard recognized or registerable qualification at present.

Although it is appreciated that other systems of pain relief and healing exist, these are not normally provided in pain clinics. They include the use of hypnosis, reflexology, homeopathy, psychic or spiritual healing, radionics, naturopathy and yoga. There is ample evidence that these alternative forms of therapy can be of help in certain cases, but it is strongly recommended that before considering them you should try to discover from a reliable source, such as the Institute for Complementary Medicine, exactly what is involved. A resource list will be found at the end of the book.

10 *Manipulative Therapy*

Some forms of manipulative therapy have been available in the United Kingdom since the beginning of the twentieth century, but until recently practitioners were, in the main, outside orthodox medicine. As a result, those who chose the services of osteopaths or chiropractors tended to feel guilty and rarely admitted to their doctor that they had resorted to what is now known as a complementary practitioner.

Over the past ten years, however, a much more open and questioning approach to all aspects of medical practice has developed, with the result that complementary medicine has become better understood and more popular. In the past the contact between orthodox and complementary medicine was very limited, but fortunately some of the barriers are now being removed. This has allowed for a useful exchange of ideas, although scope remains for much further research.

Understandably, the public has been confused by the differing views expressed about manipulation. Additionally, very few people realize that manipulators have existed among the medical profession since the early 1930s when James Mennell of St Thomas's Hospital, London, first described manipulative techniques in a book called *Backache*. By 1948, Dr James Cyriax, from the same hospital, was advocating a wider use of manipulative techniques, and eventually he began to teach the physiotherapy students at St Thomas's School of Physiotherapy how to use his techniques. Cyriax, whose concepts of orthopaedic medicine are world famous, must be credited with developing the role of the manipulative chartered physiotherapist.

In 1963 the British Association of Manipulative Medicine (B.A.M.M.) was formed to provide a forum for the increasing numbers of doctors practising manipulative techniques. The B.A.M.M.'s primary aims are to promote postgraduate education in manipulative skills and research into the subject.

It may help to understand the place of manipulation treatments available for back pain if we examine one or two of the more obvious questions.

What Is Manipulation?

The art of healing by the use of various manual pressures on the spine and its associated soft structures has been known for many centuries. In modern times the term 'mobilization' has been introduced to describe the treatment of joints which are painful or whose range of movement is restricted, by passive manual pressures, simple rhythmical motion of moderate speed and of varying magnitude. The movement thus created can be prevented by the person being treated, and the patient is therefore able to control the treatment. This enables a distinction to be made from 'manipulation', which is applied to the techniques which involve a much faster application of controlled force, which the patient cannot influence. This is often described as a high-velocity low-amplitude thrust. To avoid further confusion, 'manipulation' will be used here to encompass both techniques.

The actual techniques used by osteopaths, chiropractors and manipulative chartered physiotherapists have many similarities, as they all originate from the same ancient sources. The main variations between the three groups are in their approach to the initial clinical examination, and in their concepts of the underlying cause of the problem and of the effects of manipulation upon it.

To be effective, all manipulative techniques must be preceded by a detailed history of the pain, and by a visual and manual examination of the painful area and all other structures that may be involved. The main aim of any

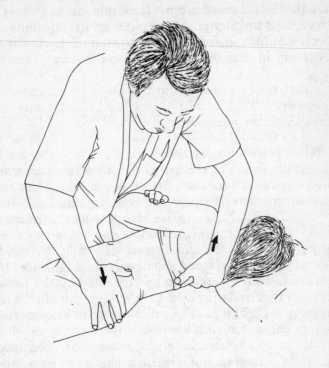

An osteopath using a sacro-iliac
thrust technique to restore
correct joint alignment

manipulative technique is to restore normal mobility to a
joint or joints where there is restricted movement and
associated dysfunction. As a result of mechanical adjust-
ments that have been made, it is also normal for there to be
a reduction in pain and muscle spasm. It is unlikely that
any manipulation will move the spinal joints more than a
small fraction of an inch, but the effects produced in the
joint capsule are believed to stimulate the mechano-
receptor organs which block painful stimuli to the brain
and produce relief.

There have been a number of research projects into the effectiveness of manipulation techniques and there seems to be no doubt that, for certain spinal problems of mechanical origin, manipulation provides a much speedier relief of pain than the other treatments used.

What is the Difference between an Osteopath, Chiropractor and Manipulative Chartered Physiotherapist?

Before considering each speciality it is important to remember that all three groups of manipulative practitioners rely on very similar techniques originating from common sources. Any major differences are likely to be found in the varying approaches to examination, diagnosis, philosophy and terminology. If, for example, you were seen in turn by a manipulative chartered physiotherapist, osteopath and chiropractor, you would find that the questions they asked might well be along similar broad lines, differing only in emphasis. The examination which followed would certainly vary as would the terminology used to explain the ultimate diagnosis. Once the treatment began it might become quite difficult to distinguish between the three specialities. Probably at present the chartered physiotherapist would be more likely to provide you with advice about prevention, perhaps even in the form of a back school, than would the osteopath or chiropractor, but this situation is changing as complementary practitioners add preventative education to their treatment programmes.

Until recently it was not possible to visit a manipulative chartered physiotherapist without first seeing a doctor, whereas anyone could seek treatment directly from an osteopath or chiropractor. This freedom was one of the attractions of osteopathy and chiropractic. In 1986 the ethical rules of the Chartered Society of Physiotherapy were revised, and as a result patients will now be able to visit a chartered physiotherapist without first seeing their doctor, although the doctor must be kept informed of the patients' progress and consulted as and when appropriate. This move should benefit both the patient and the practitioners. Once again, the importance of a thorough examination must be stressed, and the need for consultation if any untoward signs and symptoms are found.

Because manipulative therapy is a manual skill, and the systems used are essentially similar, the effectiveness of the practitioner will depend more on the skill and experience of the individual than on the particular school to which he or she belongs. In one area of the country there might be a chartered phsyiotherapist whose reputation and results were acknowledged to be first class, whilst somewhere else an osteopath or chiropractor might be in a similar position. It is not uncommon for all three groups to refer patients and to work together. It is to be hoped that as each profession begins to understand the others, there will be greater integration and co-operation.

Osteopath

The foundations of osteopathy rested on the teachings of Dr Andrew Taylor Still (1828–1917), who formulated his ideas on the treatment of disease by adjustment of the musculo-skeletal systems of the body when he became dissatisfied with the classic medical practices of his day. As a result of the success of his techniques in the mid-West of the U.S.A., the first American School of Osteopathy was founded in 1892. Since then the American osteopaths have developed into a broader profession on a par with medical doctors and, as a consequence, tend to use their traditional skills less and less, relying instead on standard medical regimes.

The influence of osteopathy was first felt in Britain in 1902, with the now-famous British School of Osteopathy being founded in 1917 by a student of Dr Still, John Martin Littlejohn. Today there are two schools of osteopathy in Britain under the direct control of the General Register of Osteopaths, in addition to the schools belonging to other osteopathic groups like the Natural Therapeutic and Osteopathic Society (N.T.O.S.) and the British Association of Manipulative Medicine (B.A.M.M.).

Students who wish to qualify as osteopathic practitioners have to undergo a four-year period of training, unless they are medical doctors or physiotherapists, who complete their course in eighteen months. On qualification, the successful students are presented with the Diploma of Osteopathy (D.O.) and if trained in the B.S.O. will be entitled to have their name placed on the general register and use the title 'Member of the Register of Osteopaths' (M.R.O.).

Many people mistakenly think that osteopathy is confined to the treatment of disorders of the back, but in fact osteopathy can be, and is, applied to any condition which can be described as a mechanical derangement. This includes restoring normal movement to joints, as well as ligaments, muscles and tendons, the release of scar tissue and adhesions and nerve entrapments, the improvement of the circulation, and reduction of swelling.

Osteopaths are trained to be able to select the type of patients who could benefit from their treatment, to identify the particular mechanical derangement(s) exhibited by the patient and then to apply their mechanical skills in order to correct and adjust the problem. The initial examination will rely heavily on a manual palpation and movement of the joints and structures involved, in order to identify areas of pain, spasm and restricted movement. These findings will then be considered in relation to the alignment and posture of the whole body and how it functions. On occasions X-rays and blood tests may be requested to aid in the formulation of a final diagnosis. Before visiting any osteopath make sure that the individual is properly qualified and also try to discover something about their reputation as a practitioner. If your local osteopath is skilled and provides results, past patients will do all the necessary 'advertising'. As a further safeguard you should check the qualifications with the B.S.O. registrar.

Chiropractor

Like osteopathy, chiropractic originated in the United States, where it was first developed in 1895 by Daniel David Palmer, a healer of some repute. The British Chiropractors' Association was established in 1925 to maintain a register of graduates from recognized colleges of chiropractic and to establish ethical standards. Virtually all of the chiropractors who practise in Britain have graduated from the Anglo-European College of Chiropractic in Bournemouth, after four years' study. The differences between osteopaths and chiropractors may not be obvious to those seeking treatment. In simple terms, chiropractors tend to concentrate on manipulations specifically of the spine in order to relieve such common problems as backache, neck pain and headaches. They use X-rays to aid diagnosis up to five times more frequently than osteopaths and also rely more on other diagnostic tests.

Should you visit a chiropractor, you will first be examined to make certain that your problem is one which can be helped. There will be the normal history-taking and examination, including tests for mobility or lack of it, and possibly an X-ray will be taken. At this stage the chiropractor will begin to concentrate on the specific problem(s), normally localized in the area of a particular spinal segment which will be identified from the earlier examinations and by touch. The usual response is to manipulate the spinal segment and possibly treat the surrounding soft structures. The number of treatment sessions necessary will depend on your response to the manipulations. If you wish to check that the chiropractor is properly qualified, look for the letters D.C. (Diploma of Chiropractic) after the name.

Manipulative Chartered Physiotherapist

The first physiotherapists to practise manipulative or mobilization techniques were students from the St Thomas's School of Physiotherapy, who were actively encouraged by the late Dr James Cyriax. By the end of the 1950s the Cyriax manipulative physiotherapists were beginning to be accepted by the hospital service, and the idea that physiotherapists could become competent in the practice of the manipulative arts gradually grew within the profession.

In the early 1960s a new system of spinal mobilization and manipulation developed by Geoffrey Maitland, an Australian physiotherapist, was introduced into Britain. The fact that this system, which contains many similarities to both the osteopathic and chiropractic techniques, became the accepted one, is attributable to the commitment and training provided by Gregory Grieve, a physiotherapy teacher and manipulative expert. Today, manipulative techniques form part of the training of all physiotherapists. However, those who wish to become expert in this form of therapy are expected to attend a course of specialized instruction and practice, either organized by or based on the curriculum developed by the Manipulative Association of Chartered Physiotherapists. This training normally takes two years' further study, in addition to the three or four years' training required to become a chartered physiotherapist (M.C.S.P.). M.A.C.P. members practise both within the National Health Service and as private physiotherapists. To be certain that a physiotherapist is chartered and also a competent manipulative practitioner, look first for the letters M.C.S.P. If your therapist has undertaken the recognized manipulative training, the letters M.A.C.P. will probably also appear after the name.

The treatment provided by your chartered physiotherapist could be very similar to that available from a chiropractor or osteopath. However, because chartered physiotherapists are also trained in electrotherapeutic techniques, massage, exercise and health education, there may be additional elements to your treatment, including greater emphasis on preventative measures and advice about posture and methods of body-use in work and leisure activities.

As a matter of principle, it is wise not to seek treatment from more than one practitioner at any one time. This will increase the difficulties of those who are trying to treat you, and is unlikely to be beneficial. It is not easy to give specific advice as to which form of therapy would suit your particular problem, because there are so many variable factors, but it is hoped that the details provided here will give some guidance in helping you to come to a decision.

To Sum Up ...

Back pain has proved to be a baffling problem for the human species and one for which, over a long period of time, there have been explanations and 'cures' beyond number. Our present knowledge about the back and its disorders is growing steadily, and as a result some solutions are emerging, but it is still true that more is known about the apparent cause and development of disease and injury to the spine than about the ways in which to relieve the pain that so often accompanies it.

It is a fact that many episodes of back pain occur as a result of fairly minor events related to faulty posture, prolonged and repeated stress and incorrect use of the spinal mechanism. If advice and treatment were sought for these problems at their onset, in a large number of cases a positive cure could be achieved and further injury prevented. Unfortunately, far too frequently these minor irritant episodes are ignored in the hope that they will go away, as often they do, only to return again and again. Eventually, a major episode of back pain may result, and by this time a full and proper cure may not be possible.

The solution to the persistent problem of back pain is the equal responsibility of the individual and of those who practise healing, be they classified as orthodox or complementary. A healthy respect for the body together with a better understanding of its workings are essential before we can really begin to beat back pain. Without a personal commitment to self-health and self-help by individuals, no system devised by health practitioners can hope to have a lasting effect.

Whilst those who practise medicine and allied therapies need to look at themselves and the help they provide in a constructively critical manner, the potential sufferer can do much to improve the system that currently exists. If the general public began to ask about back care and the many alternatives that are available, it is likely that this would stimulate practitioners to take a wider view in their approach to those they sought to treat. Gradually, armed with a reasonable level of knowledge, the back pain sufferer would become able to help him- or herself more, and when necessary to make a more informed choice about the best source of assistance.

Finally, if the complex physical and mental aspects of the problem we loosely refer to as back pain are to be resolved, the narrow, limited concepts of the past will have to be discarded. In their place there will have to be a broader-based system of prevention and healing. There is a wealth of knowledge available today, but it is scattered like an unassembled jigsaw. All of us who claim to have an interest in healing – sufferer and curer alike – must work to combine our pieces of the jigsaw in order to arrive at a more finished picture.

Back pain can be beaten, let us do it together!

Resource List

General

Back Pain Association
Grundy House
31–33 Park Road
Teddington
Middlesex

Ergonomics Society
University of Technology
Loughborough
Leics LE11 3TU

National Bedding Federation Ltd
251 Brompton Road
London SW3 2EZ

Orthodox

British Medical Association
British Medical Association House
Tavistock Square
London WC1H 9JP

General Medical Council
44 Hallam Street
London W1N 6AE

Institute of Orthopaedics
234 Great Portland Street
London WC1N 5HG

*The Arthritis and Rheumatism Council for Research
(formerly British Arthritis and Rheumatism Council)*
Faraday House
8–10 Charing Cross Road
London WC1H OHN

Chartered Society of Physiotherapy
14 Bedford Row
London NW3 5AU

Institute of Orthopaedic Medicine
81 Belsize Lane
London NW3 5AU

Organisation of Chartered Physiotherapists in Private Practice
c/o 14 Bedford Row
London WC1R 4ED

Manipulative Therapy

Manipulative Association of Chartered Physiotherapists
c/o 14 Bedford Row
London WC1R 4ED

British Association of Manipulative Medicine
22 Wimpole Street
London W1M 7AD

The Natural Therapeutic and Osteopathic Society and Register
14 Windsor Road
Bexleyheath
Kent

General Council and Register of Osteopaths
16 Buckingham Gate
London SW1E 6LB

Anglo-European College of Chiropractic
Cavendish Road
Bournemouth BH1 1RA

Complementary Therapies

Society of Teachers of the Alexander Technique
10 London House
266 Fulham Road
London SW10 9EL

British Acupuncture Association and Register Ltd
34 Alderney Street
London SW1V 4EU

Traditional Acupuncture Society
St Albans House
Portland Street
Royal Leamington Spa
Warwickshire CV32 5EZ

British Medical Acupuncture Association
15 Devonshire Place
London W1N 1PB

For information on Psychic Healing, Radiesthesia, Homeo-pathy, Naturopathy and Yoga send SAE for details of your local practitioners to:

The Institute for Complementary Medicine
21 Portland Place
London W1N 3AF

Book List

Anderson, T. McClurg (1951). *Human Kinetics and Analysing Body Movements*, William Heinemann Medical Books, London.

Anderson, T. McClurg (1970). 'Housework with Ease', pub. The Scottish Council of Physical Recreation.

Anon. 'Prospectus of the Anglo-European College of Chiropractic', Parkwood Road, Bournemouth.

Anon. 'Back Care', pub. Health Education Bureau of Ireland.

Anon. 'Osteopathy and the Register', pub. General Council and Register of Osteopaths Ltd, 16 Buckingham Gate, London SW1E 6LB.

Anon. (1979). 'You and the Way You Sit', pub. Accident Compensation Commission, Wellington, New Zealand.

Barker, S. (1981). *The Revolutionary Way to Use Your Body for Total Energy – The Alexander Technique*. Bantam Books Inc., New York.

Barlow, W. (1984). *The Alexander Principle*, Arrow Books Ltd, London.

Byway, C., Fletcher, B., Hayne, C. R. (1980). 'Fight Back – A Self Help Programme for Back Pain Sufferers', pub. Spencer (Banbury) Ltd, Banbury, Oxon. OX16 8DP.

Corlett, N., Wilson, J., Manenica, I., (1986). *The Ergonomics of Working Postures*, Taylor and Francis, London.

Crawshaw, C., Frazer, A. M., Merriam, W. F., Mulholland, R. C., Webb, J. K., (1984). 'A Comparison of Surgery with Chymopapain in the Treatment of Sciatica', *Spine*, vol. 9, no. 2, pp. 195–8.

Cyriax, J. H. and Cyriax, P. J., (1984). 'The Illustrated Manual of Orthopaedic Medicine', prepared for Geigy Pharmaceuticals, England.

Delvin, D. (1975). 'You and Your Back', pub. Back Pain Association, London.

Deyo, R. A., Diehl, A. K., Rosenthal, M. (1986). 'How Many Days of Bed Rest for Acute Low Back Pain? – A Randomised Clinical Trial', *The New England Journal of Medicine*, vol. 315, no. 17, pp. 1064–70.

Di Fabio, R. P., (1986). 'Clinical Assessment of Manipulation and Mobilisation of the Lumbar Spine – A Critical Review of the Literature', *Physical Therapy*, vol. 66, no. 1., Jan., pp. 51–3.

Dove, C. I., (1983). 'Osteopathy', *Midwife, Health Visitors and Community Nurse*, vol. 19, September.

Fahrni, W. H. and Trueman, G. E., (1965). 'Comparative Radiological Study of the Spines of a Primitive Population with North Americans and Northern Europeans', *Journal of Bone and Joint Surgery*, vol. 47B, August.

Fahrni, W. H., (1975). 'Conservative Treatment of Lumbar Disc Degeneration: Our Primary Responsibility', *Ortho Clinics of North America*, vol. 6, Jan., pp. 93–103.

Fenton, J. V., (1973). *Choice of Habit – Poise, Free Movement and the Practical Use of the Body*, MacDonalds & Evans Ltd.

Finneson, B. E., (1981). *Low Back Pain*, J.B. Lippincott Co., Philadelphia.

Frankel, V. H. and Nordin, M. (1980). *Basic Biomechanics of the Skeletal System*, Lea and Febiger, Philadelphia.

Grandjean, E. (1980). *Fitting the Task to the Man – An Ergonomic Approach*, Taylor and Francis Ltd, London.

Grandjean, E., Hunting, W. and Nishiyma (1984). 'Preferred VDT Workstation Settings, Body Posture and Physical Impairments', *Applied Ergonomics*, vol. 15, no. 2, June.

Handley, J. (1987). 'Back to Basic Body-Use in Physical Education', pub. Education Department, London Borough of Enfield.

Hartman, L. S. (1985). *Handbook of Osteopathic Technique*, Hutchinson & Co. Ltd, London.

Hayne, C. R. (1980). 'Acute Back Care', pub. Spencer (Banbury) Ltd, Banbury, Oxon. OX16 8DP.

Hayne, C. R. (1986). 'Prophylaxis and Ergonomic Considerations' in *Modern Manual Therapy of the Vertebral Column*, ed. Grieve, G. P., Churchill Livingstone, Edinburgh.

Inglis, B. (1978). *The Book of the Back*, Ebury Press, London.

Jaffe, M. and Cooper, S. (1985). *Get Your Back in Shape*, Thorsons Publishers Ltd, Wellingborough, Northants.

Jayson, M. I. (1980). *The Lumbar Spine and Back Pain*, Pitman Medical, London.

Kapandji, I. A. (1985). *The Physiology of the Joints*, vol. 3, *The Trunk and Vertebral Column*, Churchill Livingstone, Edinburgh.

Keim, H. A. and Kirkaldy-Willis, W. H. (1980). 'Low Back Pain – Clinical Symposia', vol. 32, no. 6, pub. CIBA Pharmaceutical Co.

McKenzie, R. A. (1984). 'The Lumbar Spine – Mechanical Diagnosis and Therapy', pub. Spinal Publications Ltd, P.O. Box 2, Waikanae, New Zealand.

MacNab, I. (1973). 'Backache', pub. The Workmen's Compensation Board, Ontario, Canada.

Mandal, A. C. (1985). *The Seated Man – Homo Sedens*, Dafnia Publications, Taarbek, Strandvej 49, 2930 Klampenborg, Denmark.

Michel, T. H. (1985). *Pain – International Perspectives in Physical Therapy*, Churchill Livingstone, Edinburgh.

Nachemson, A. L. and Elfstrom, G. (1970). 'Intravital Dynamic Pressure Measurements in Lumbar Discs. A Study of Common Movements Manoeuvres and Exercises', *Scan. J. Rehab Med.* 2 (Suppl.1.), pp. 1–40.

Nachemson, A. L. (1976). 'The Lumbar Spine: an Orthopaedic Challenge', *Spine*, vol. 1, pp. 59–71.

Paterson, J. K. and Burn, L. (1985). *An Introduction to Medical Manipulation*, MTP Press Ltd, Lancaster.

Pheasant, S. T. (1984). 'Anthropometrics – An Introduction for Schools and Colleges', pub. British Standards Institute, London.

Pope, M. H., Frymoyer, J. W., Andersson, G. (1984). *Occupational Low Back Pain*, Praeger Publishers, New York.

Porter, R. W. (1983). *Understanding Back Pain*, Patient Handbook 13, Churchill Livingstone, Edinburgh.

Stoddard, A. (1980). *The Back – Relief from Pain*, Martin Dunitz Ltd, London.

Tichauer, E. R. (1976). 'Biomechanics Sustains Occupational Health'. *Industrial Engineer*, vol. 8, pp. 46–56.

Wells, N. (1985). 'Back Pain', no. 78 in a Series on Health Problems, Office of Health Economics, 12 Whitehall, London SW1A 2DY. (Useful source of Back Pain statistics.)

Index

Abdominal muscles, 15
Acupuncture, 119–21
Acute back pain, 40–42
Age, ageing, 3, 8, 24
Alexander, F. Matthias, 78
Alexander technique, 77–9
Alternative therapy, 1, 121
Anaesthetist, 98
Anderson, T. McClurg, 53
Assessment, functional, 109–10

Back pain
   acute, 40–42
   chronic, 26–7
   gynaecological, 27–8
   inflammatory, 28–9
   investigations for, 98–102
   mild, 36
   reactions to, 29–31
   survival, 40–43
Back school, 110–12
Beds
   buying guide, 70–73
   getting out of, 69
   making, 52
Bowden, Ruth E. M., xi
British Association of
   Manipulative Medicine
   (B.A.M.M.), 110
British School of
   Osteopathy, 126

Canal, spinal, 7

Car seats, 63–4
CAT scan, 102
Causes of back pain,
   common, 18ff
Cervical spine, 9–10
Chemonucleolysis, 106–7
Chest region, 10
Chiropractic, chiropractors,
   128
      Anglo-European
         College of, 128
Chronic back pain, 26–7
Chymopapain, 106–7
Clinic, pain, 115–16
Clinical examination, 100
Coccyx, 11
Cold therapy, 36–8
Consultant, hospital, 97–8
Cord, spinal, 7, 16–17
Cyriax, James 129

Degeneration, 8
Diagnostic ultrasound, 102
Disc lesions, acute, 23–6
Discogram, 101

Easing mild back pain, 36–40
Education, 110
Electrical relief for back
   pain, 116–18
Ergonomics, 110
Examination, clinical, 100
Exercise, 80–90
      routine I, 82–4

routine II, 84–5
    routine III, 85–7
    supplementary, 87–90

Facet joints, 7–8
    injuries to, 21–2
Family doctor, 95–6
'Fibrositis', 19
Forsell, M. Z., 110
Functional assessment,
    109–10
Furniture, selection, 64–5
Fusion, spinal, 104–5

Gall bladder, 2
Gardening, 52, 91–2
General practitioner, 95–6
Grieve, Gregory, 129
Gynaecological back pain,
    27–8

Handling loads, 53–6
Heat therapy, 37, 38
Help
    medical, 95ff
    self-, 32ff
Hormonal activity, effects
    of, 23
Hospital consultant, 97–8

Inflammation,
    inflammatory processes,
    2, 28–9
Injections for back pain,
    116
Injuries
    facet joint, 21–22
    soft tissue, 18–20
    spinal, 21–6
Intervertebral discs, 4, 6, 8
    ruptures of, 23–4

Investigations for back
  pain, 98–102

Joint capsules, 8
    in inflammatory
      conditions, 28

Kidney stones, 2
Kinetic handling, 53

Laboratory tests, 102
Laminectomy, 105
Leisure activities, 91–4
Lifting, 53–6
Ligaments, 6, 12–13, 27
    effect of hormonal
      activity on, 23
    in inflammatory
      conditions, 28
    injuries to, 19–20
Littlejohn, J. M., 126
Loads, handling, 53–6
Lumbago, 1
Lumbar spine, 3

Maitland, Geoffrey, 129
Manipulation, 122–9
Manipulative chartered
  physiotherapist, 125
Mandal, A.C., 62
Massage, 39–40
Mechanical stress, 2, 3
Mennell, James, 122
Mild back pain, easing,
    36–40
Muscles
    abdominal, 15
    spinal, 6, 13–15
    strains, 19
    strength and tone, 80
Myelogram, 101

National Back Pain
  Association, xi, 77, 133
National Therapeutic and
  Osteopathic Society
  (N.T.O.S.), 127
Neck, 9–10
Nerves, 7
Nerve roots, 16–17
Neurologist, 97
Neurosurgeon, 97

Orthopaedic surgeon, 97
Osteopath, osteopathy,
  126–7
    British School of, 126
    London School of
      (N.T.O.S.), 127

Pain
    chart, 34
    clinic, 115–16
    electrical relief for,
      116–18
    pregnancy and, 23,
      27–8
    receptors, 2
    scale, 35
    transmission of, 2
    types and causes of, 18ff
Palmer, D.D., 128
Patient-Administered
  Subjective Evaluation
  (P.A.S.E.), 109
Physiotherapy, chartered
  physiotherapist, 108–15
    examination, 109
    manipulative, 125,
      128–9
    treatment, 110
Post-operative routines,
  105–6

Posture, 44 ff
    control of, 46–8
    ideal, 45–6
    pregnancy and, 27–8
    sitting, 57–65
    standing, 48–50
Pregnancy and back pain,
  23, 27–8
Psychiatrist, 98

Reactions to back pain,
  29–31
Recovery, chances of, 30
Relaxation, 73–7
Rheumatologist, 97
Resource list, 133–5
Routines, post-operative,
  105–6

Sacrum, 4, 11
Sacro-iliac strains, 22–3
Sciatica, 1
Seats, car, 63–4
Self-assessment, 32ff
    questionnaire, 33–5
Sexual intercourse, 93
Sitting, 57–61
    at work, 61–3
Sleep, 66
Sleeping positions, 66–8
Spinal
    canal, 7
    cord, 7, 16–17
    fusion, 104–5
    injuries, 216
    muscles, 6, 13–15
    problems, 9ff
    supports, 42–3, 112–15
    surgery, 103–6
Spine
    and ageing, 6

cervical, 9–10
function of, 3
general view of, 3–9
lumbar, 3
movements, 4
thoracic, 10
Sports and back pain, 92
Standing at work, 50
Stooping, 50–3
Still, A. T., 126
Strains
muscular, 19
sacro-iliac, 22–3
Stress, mechanical, 2, 3
Supports, spinal, 42–3,
112–15
Surgery, spinal, 103–6
Surviving acute back pain,
40–42

TENS, 117–18
Thorax, thoracic spine, 10
Types of back pain,
common, 18ff

Ultrasound, diagnostic,
102

Vertebrae, 4, 6–7
Vibration, 38–9

Working
in a standing position,
50
in a sitting position,
61–3

X-ray, 100